MENOPAUSE

Let's get to the point, period.

**A Self-Care Book for Women to Manage Their
Menopausal Symptoms, Optimize Their Emotional
Health and Embrace this Transition**

SUSAN MINIHANE

Printed Worldwide
First Printing 2023
First Edition 2023

10 9 8 7 6 5 4 3 2 1

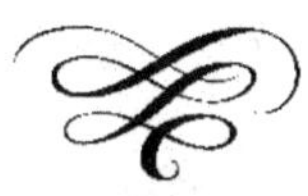

*For my daughters, Lauren and Caroline, who made
PMS and visits from Aunt Flo worth it.*

TABLE OF CONTENTS

FOREWORD

I see you. You are not invisible. You are not alone. If you are reading this book, you are either going through menopause or have a loved one who is. I wrote this book for you. We live in a time where we have so much information at our fingertips yet so many of us are still in the dark about menopause.

My menopausal journey began five years ago. After a routine yearly physical and full blood panel, my doctor called me to share the results. Luckily, my tests returned normal, but he casually mentioned that I had gone through menopause. Wait…what?! I was driving my car at the time and literally pulled over as I was so taken back by this news. I asked him how he knew, and he said that he tested my hormone levels with my full panel blood test, just to check given my age.

Anger aside, I was 48 at the time and shocked by this news. It was an unexpected blow to my ego. I drove home feeling bewildered and a bit devastated. While I didn't want to have any more children, I didn't want to be "old." You may wonder how I didn't know that I had gone through menopause. Well, I had a Mirena IUD at the time, so I no longer had monthly periods just sporadic bleeding. My doctor said I was lucky that I had sailed through menopause as he had many female patients with all sorts of menopausal issues that were having a difficult time.

Who were these patients and why weren't they talking? I thought about his comment and considered it more and realized that my friends don't discuss menopause either. We discuss life, our families, books, food, and everything under else under the sun but menopause seems taboo. This is a sad and stark contrast to when I was a girl and my friends and I couldn't wait to get our periods. It meant we were now women! We were cool. We were mature. The school nurse spoke to us about menstruation. The biggest worry was how and when our first period would arrive. Would it be privately at home or publicly and embarrassingly during gym class or at the pool, or while wearing white pants? So much excitement and intrigue and anticipation. Some of us carried a pretty pencil case filled with pads and wondered when we would finally get to unzip the bag and use its' contents.

Unfortunately, this excitement and anticipation does not happen with menopause. While we should be thrilled about no longer having PMS and monthly bleeding, most women I know seem to endure this stage of life quietly and resentfully. Perhaps we complain about insomnia, hot flashes, weight gain, and other menopausal symptoms, there is no school nurse nor mother handing out a book or friend excited for you to go through this change of life.

After I learned that I had gone through menopause, I decided to have my IUD removed. Soon after, I started to experience insomnia, hot flashes, psoriasis, aches, and pains. I met with a new female doctor and was told it was just another aspect of menopause. Again, I wondered what was going on?! I had already gone through menopause two years prior. She mentioned that women can have symptoms post menopause. Again, I was very confused.

I turned to Dr. Google, as you do, and sought out articles and books on the subject. Some books were pro hormone replacement therapy ("HRT") while others were anti- HRT. Some books mentioned alternative therapies and nonconventional methods to manage the transition. However, most books I looked at seemed to have an agenda, whether it be medical interventions or natural therapies. I am a busy person and wanted the cliff notes; the so called "takeaways" of this curious stage of my life with a broad perspective. I couldn't find this, so I did my research and worked with consultants to write this book. It is much longer than an online article or blog post yet comprehensive and open minded to both HRT and alternative therapies. As a proponent of living a healthy lifestyle, I have also included exercises and foods that may benefit women going through this transition.

I wish that I had a book like this five years ago when my doctor gave me the results of my blood tests. I would have had the facts and information needed to understand what was going on in my body and make decisions on how best to better navigate through this inevitable part of life. So here it is, and I hope it'll help you.

February 2023

INTRODUCTION

As women, we go through two major physiological transitions in our lives: puberty and menopause. While the curtain has been peeled back when it comes to puberty and what to expect, menopause remains somewhat a mystery—with many women not knowing much about this time until they're in the midst of their transition (or, in my case, past it). Yet, in many circles, menopause is referred to as a "second puberty." But where puberty is celebrated and dubbed a time where we truly *become* a "woman," menopause is swept under the rug. But here's the thing: Like that dust and dirt under the rug that you're trying to avoid, ignoring menopause isn't going to make it go away. In fact, not acknowledging that menopause eventually happens to every woman is setting many of us up for months and *years* of strife and confusion. All of a sudden, our bodies have a mind of their own. Cold one minute, hot the next. Menopause is a force to be reckoned with. Sometimes, it's even hard to recognize if these changes and symptoms are brought on by menopause or simply life itself. Yet another chicken or egg dilemma, so to speak.

At the end of the day, menopause is a journey that not only women go on but their families and spouses or partners do too. To travel in harmony, we need to learn how to understand the physical and mental challenges we face during menopause, so that we can maintain positive relationships with those we care about the most and enter this new chapter of life with ease. So, how can we make this journey that much easier and arrive still feeling like "us"? Undeniably, this can be challenging, and many women struggle along the way. During this time, it's important that we reach out and find the help we need. Self-help and self-care are both important factors when it comes to tackling the menopausal transition.

So, in this book, we will explore menopause in more detail. How can we better prepare? What can we do to make this transitional time *easier*? And how can we break down those menopausal barriers and taboos? Well, it all starts with talking about it.

While some women will sail through menopause without many issues, other women experience it in a more traumatic way, whether that be physically, mentally, or both. Within these pages, we will explore the various menopausal treatments and remedies available, as well as look at exercise and nutrition that can be beneficial to women during this stage of life. Not all is lost! And no, menopause isn't the end of your life. In fact, it's only just the beginning of a brand-new era. So, ladies, let's grab the bull by the horns, so to speak. It's time to take charge and own this part of your life, while stepping forward into that next phase and on to a fresh page.

CHAPTER ONE

WHAT REALLY IS MENOPAUSE?

"Did you know that the average age that a woman enters natural menopause is 52, though the transition can start as early as 40 or as late as 60?"

– Strive Health

Just like its symptoms, menopause is not clearly defined. Perhaps, the problem is that menopause is not a single event in a woman's life. We often think of puberty as a single event—when a girl gets her period and begins menstruation. Voila! It's happened. But there's always more to it than that. Puberty consists of different stages. There's the varying awkward and exciting phases of growth, such as the defining moment of getting your first bra. In many ways, it is very similar to menopause. Yet, instead of "everything" starting up as it is with puberty, menopause can somewhat best be described as the reverse; everything is slowing down.

Menopause consists of three different stages: perimenopause, menopause, and post menopause. All bodies are different and for some women, they go through these three stages fast. Meanwhile, others experience it over the course of 10+ years. Just like in puberty and pregnancy, every woman will have her own experience with menopause.

In this book, we are going to elaborate on all three of these stages. First, let's try to define the word "menopause" in the medical sense.

According to the Merriam-Webster dictionary, "menopause is the natural cessation of menstruation that usually occurs between the ages of 45 and 55." Menopause is actually a French word (That fact alone might make us see it in a slightly different light!) and was first used in 1822. It is commonly referred to as "the change of life."

Dictionary aside, if you have not had a period for one year, most doctors would say you are in the postmenopausal stage, and this is often how the time of menopause is defined.

All in all, menopause usually takes place between the ages of 45 and 55, but there are many factors that may cause women to experience an early onset of menopause. These factors include medical treatments, surgery, and nutrition.

In fact, hormonal changes and imbalances take place many years before menopause has occurred. This is often referred to as "perimenopause."

Problems and health conditions that may occur at the onset of or during menopause can include several or many symptoms, such as hot flashes, insomnia, body aches, joint pain, skin issues, brain fog, weight gain, decreased sex drive, emotional difficulties, digestive disorders, fatigue, and weakened eyesight.

While some women may only have a few symptoms, other women have every symptom under the sun. For example, I had a friend whose first symptom was itchy skin. She could not understand why she suddenly started to experience itchy skin. She was baffled. Her doctor was baffled. Despite tests, medical appointments, and trying various skin lotions, no one could pinpoint the answer as to "why." That was until she visited a naturopath who understood what was going on and explained that in the menopausal stage of a woman's life, hormonal imbalances and circulatory problems can cause your skin to itch (I had no idea either!). You may not have a rash, but it can feel like something is crawling on your skin any make it itchy. Not exactly what most people think of when they hear the word "menopause."

Another friend of mine thought she might have arthritis; she was very active and healthy but woke up most mornings with sore muscles and joints. She went to the doctor and had blood tests for rheumatoid arthritis, but her results showed that she was normal so, her doctor ended up attributing these aches and pains to menopause. It definitely makes you wonder why these kinds of symptoms happen. The truth? The reasons aren't entirely clear, but inflammation seems to play a big part.

Luckily, there are many medical and natural treatments available to make the journey through menopause that much easier. However, every woman's body is different and has different symptoms. Hence, these treatments are not a one-size-fits-all approach.

When you are going through the various stages of menopause, you must take a pragmatic approach and find out what works for you. This could be through trial and error. Perhaps, hormone replacement therapy will work for you, but then again, many women benefit from natural remedies such as supplements and homeopathy. Sometimes, a combination of the two may be best.

In this book, we are going to cover medical treatments, natural remedies, movement, and nutrition. It is important to stay open-minded. Also, YOU need to be proactive and prepared to take the necessary steps to make your menopausal journey better. If you don't get involved, your body will take charge of you instead! Don't be afraid to seek out advice from health care professionals, friends, and women that you trust. Don't shy away from discussing menopause. It's about time we did!

CHAPTER TWO

THE STAGES OF MENOPAUSE

"Menopause is like a rollercoaster ride - one minute you're up, the next you're down, and you're never quite sure when it's going to end."

- Unknown

Ah, the stages of menopause! For many women, the problem here is that there does not seem to be a very clear borderline as to when they transition from one stage to the next. Put bluntly, more research is needed to truly understand and define these stages further. So, let's dig a little deeper into these different menopausal stages. What is the current knowledge regarding the stages of menopause? What happens at each stage? What common symptoms may occur?

PERIMENOPAUSE

Until recently, no one was talking about perimenopause. This is the first menopausal stage women experience before they go through the "actual" menopause. In other words, it's pre-menopause. During this time, you'll still be ovulating (perhaps somewhat irregularly) and have some form of period (also likely somewhat irregularly). And yes, you can get pregnant and still need to use some form of birth control if you don't want to have a baby.

When perimenopause begins is hard to define and is unique to every woman. Generally, perimenopause can start any time between the ages of 37 and 50. By the time most women reach age 50, they have experienced some or many symptoms that are associated with perimenopause. The most common symptom, as referenced above, is erratic periods. This happens whether you are on a contraceptive pill or using another form of hormonal birth control. As your hormonal balance starts to change, so does your body's response to hormonal birth control and your flow can vary.

There are blood tests you can take to check your hormone levels, like I did. Estrogen and progesterone are the two most important hormones in the female body that regulate the function of the uterus (More about these two hormones later in this book). Doctors can test these hormone levels with a blood test, giving you some insight into what is going on. Another common test performed to determine hormonal levels is the DUTCH test, which uses urine and saliva as opposed to blood samples.

It is important to note that there are problems with these tests as the balance of your hormones shifts rapidly; one day your estrogen levels may be up, the next day, progesterone and other hormones like cortisol will take over. In other words, your hormones take on a bit of a rollercoaster ride, making it hard to pinpoint what exactly is going on. To truly determine if you are experiencing perimenopause, it is best to go by the symptoms.

Symptoms of perimenopause include:

* Erratic periods

* Hot flashes

* Weight gain

* Fatigue

* Loss of libido

* Thinning hair or change in hair quality

* Irregular heartbeat

* Headaches and migraines

* Dry skin

* Bloating

* Aches and pains

* Change in eyesight

However, this is not the end of the list. Some women can experience other symptoms which may not be included here. And the unfortunate truth is that these symptoms can be both exhausting and frightening. There are a wide range of symptoms can be attributed to other ailments as well. Thus, a trip down the rabbit hole with Dr. Google can definitely leave you feeling a bit shaken up. Remember, knowledge is power here! Whether you're currently going through perimenopause or have already gone through menopause, knowing all of this information can help you navigate this time of life better.

To make this transitional period easier for women, more research *is* needed. Doctors and scientists need to develop a better understanding of why these symptoms and health conditions present themselves during perimenopause. The prevailing theory is that hormonal imbalances lead to inflammatory responses in the body. But, again, this isn't well understood. With more and more research coming out every day, hopefully soon, we'll have better insights into what happens as a woman's body enters menopause.

MENOPAUSE

Don't assume for one minute that your period will magically stop when you turn 50 (As much as many of us may wish our period away and with as little fuss as possible!). Many women actually have their period until they are much older. Everyone is different. Your age of menopause is often based on your genetics, that is, it is related to when your mother went through menopause. Another reason some women experience menopause later in life is because of environmental factors. In some countries, hormones are added to livestock feed to fatten up cows, pigs, chicken, lamb, etc. These hormones are then passed down the food chain. So when we eat the food, we also digest the hormones in the meat which will, in turn, affect us during menopause. That old cliche saying "You are what you eat" isn't far from the truth.

Some perimenopausal symptoms may further persist into menopause. On the other hand, certain symptoms may reduce when you reach menopause. Yet, either way, you are likely to experience physical effects. On top of that, don't be surprised if you experience emotional effects as well. Depression and anxiety are common when you reach menopause and your hormonal balance changes.

But this doesn't mean you need to fear the worst! Many women find great joy and transformation during this time in their life. After decades of PMS, monthly periods, and practicing safe sex, they are finally free and may feel truly liberated. On top of this, around this time, many parents experience their children leaving the home for the first time. They may also experience changes in their career or relationships, leading to the start of a new era.

If you have had a hysterectomy, your body often skips perimenopausal symptoms altogether and goes straight to the actual menopause, which for some women can be traumatic and for other women, it might be quick and easy. Again, every woman's experience of menopause is different and unique.

POSTMENOPAUSE

Once you have "gone through menopause," symptoms and physical effects of the menopausal stage of your life *should* get better. You may wonder if this is always the case but again, it really depends on the individual. Some women are symptom-free for years, but then experience hot flashes or joint pain suddenly, as I did.

What is happening in your life can also affect your postmenopausal experience. If you are under a lot of stress or anxiety, symptoms that you've been experiencing during perimenopause and actual menopause may persist. In these situations, finding ways to tackle your stress is imperative (more on this later).

Now... here's a big one: Will you feel older after menopause? This was my initial gut reaction. I thought, 'Menopause?! I'm old!' This was immediately followed by, 'I don't want to be old!' But age truly is just a number. While some women say they feel older, other women have a different view. They say they feel rejuvenated and free as they no longer worry about monthly periods nor getting pregnant. Women who've had children earlier in life may feel happier as their kids are older and more independent, so they now have more time for themselves and their own needs. The moral of the story here? It all comes down to your own mindset and perspective. Again, life doesn't end with menopause nor should it.

And although you may experience physical and mental symptoms during menopause, you can try combating them with HRT, alternative therapies, diet, and exercise which we will discuss more later in this book.

Remember, the stages of menopause are not an illness nor disease. The best way to view it is as a natural transition. Perhaps even a new era. A fresh page. The closing of one chapter and the start of another.

CHAPTER THREE

HOW MENOPAUSE AFFECTS YOUR BODY

"All great changes are preceded by chaos."
- Deepak Chopra

In any stage of life, our physical state impacts our mental state, and vice versa. Menopause affects women both mentally and physically. The truth is that no part of the body is left unaffected by menopause. After all, our hormones drive most processes within the body and influence how we feel.

The internal effects of menopause are on the uterus and ovaries where the two key hormones, estrogen, and progesterone, regulate the female reproduction system. As these hormones levels start to fluctuate during perimenopause, you may experience both physical and mental changes. Some may be more subtle while others will be more noticeable. If you have had a hysterectomy, then you have experienced what doctors call "surgical menopause."

So, what's going on beneath the surface? Why are we feeling some kind of way during this transitional time?

ERRATIC OVULATION LEADS TO ERRATIC PERIODS

Erratic ovulation is common during the menopausal years. One month you may have a period and the next month you may skip it and not have a period at all. Some women go months without a period and then suddenly, they have periods closer together. Periods may be longer or shorter than usual and bleeding can be heavier or lighter than usual. A couple of months later, they may flip and become normal again. In many ways, "usual" and "normal" periods become a figment of our imagination. This can be both confusing and frustrating, especially if you had a lifetime of regular monthly cycles. Inevitably, our body becomes an unpredictable entity which can be exhausting in multiple ways. But, again, this is temporary. Eventually, you will come out of the other side, period-free.

At the same time, if you notice any changes that concern you, it is best to visit a doctor. If you don't already, you may want to see a female doctor. She may have already gone through menopause and if she hasn't, she will still have a more vested interest in your experience as she has the undeniable trait of being female too.

HEAVY PERIODS

As hormonal levels change, some women experience heavy periods, referred to as menorrhagia, during perimenopause. One side effect of heavy periods is anemia; a lack of iron and sometimes other B vitamins.

Obvious signs of anemia are being tired, bruising easily, and pale skin. Thus, paying extra attention to your diet and getting enough iron is important. Depending on your choice of diet, red meat and/or dark green leafy vegetables are easy ways to combat anemia. Your doctor may recommend an iron or vitamin B supplement. Also, make sure your diet contains plenty of vitamin C (Grab a glass of orange juice or a handful of strawberries to obtain the recommended daily value of this vitamin!) which helps with the absorption of iron and vitamin B.

PAINFUL PERIODS

Dysmenorrhea is the medical name for painful periods. For many women, unfortunately, painful periods are common. They can leave you feeling sick and even bedridden. While many experience painful periods and cramps during their prime menstruating years, the bad news is that it doesn't always end. Some continue to experience cramps and pain or even *begin* to experience painful periods in their menopausal years. The reason is not clearly understood, but fluctuating hormonal levels is the likely suspect. As estrogen levels in the body drop, women experience more inflammation which can lead to a higher chance of experiencing painful periods. Another factor to consider is the build-up of the uterine lining. During menopause, it can get thicker and lead to heavy and painful periods (and maybe not exactly the day you had planned).

BLOATING

A variety of physical reasons are responsible for bloating. As your periods become further apart, the lining of the uterus becomes thicker. This may lead to bloating, as well as problems with digestion (just when we think things couldn't get worse).

Changing hormone levels during menopause can cause your body to retain water and also slow down your digestion process which can also lead to this less-than-desirable bloat. Yes, it might seem as though your body has a mind of its own! But bear with me. We will eventually get to what you can do about all of this, helping you take back control of your body and this time in your life.

THE MYSTERY OF HOT FLASHES

One minute you're too cold. The next, you're far too hot. It's like someone turned your internal furnace on overdrive (without consulting or asking you first!). Hot flashes are one of the many mysteries surrounding menopause, and one of the biggest complaints from many women.

In other bad news… Despite research into hot flashes, scientists have *not* found a conclusive solution. But here is what we do know: Your body has its own thermostat. It is called the hypothalamus. The theory goes that decreased estrogen makes this internal thermostat more sensitive to temperature changes. Thus, during menopause, your body can get too hot and a "hot flash" is produced. It's almost like a released safety valve. On top of this, many women experience more hot flashes at night when they are in bed (also called "night sweats"). This means that once cozy and heavy comforter or blanket might just be too much for many women during this stage of their lives. Cotton bedding and light pyjamas are the best way forward (or even sleeping naked! I'm not kidding. For some, sleeping naked can even reduce stress and anxiety.). More advice on how to deal with hot flashes will be explored later in this book. Hang in there!

THINNING OF THE BONES

Many women are prone to osteoporosis when they go through menopause. Osteoporosis is when your bones become thin and brittle because your skeleton is absorbing less calcium. Symptoms of osteoporosis are skeletal aches, feeling tired, and some women may have dental health problems, such as loose teeth. Yes, you read that right! Osteoporosis causes the bone in your gums to thin, leading to the potential loosening of the teeth.

Although we know more about osteoporosis, it's still a health condition that is not fully understood. There are more than just hormones involved as osteoporosis affects both men and women. Eating calcium-rich food is undeniably important. Exercising in the right way also helps; resistance training and light aerobic workouts are both important in building and strengthening our bones and body (which is why you may see many in the health space encouraging perimenopause, menopausal, and post-menopausal women to go lift some weights on a regular basis! No, ladies, lifting won't make you bulky. Quite the opposite actually. On top of the benefits for our bones, it also has immense advantages when it comes to our metabolism and maintaining a healthy weight. More on this later in this book.).

VAGINAL DRYNESS

Let's not be shy; many women feel sore, dry, and itchy around their vagina during menopause. This can result in painful sex, frequent urination, and lead to urinary tract infections. And as embarrassing as this may feel to discuss, it's all too real for many women, even interfering with their daily lives and relationships.

Luckily, you can buy lubricants at your local drug store to deal with dryness. Some women say that more foreplay helps as well, while others claim that sex toys can solve the problem. Ultimately, you've got to find what works for you!

The solution is often a personal one and trying a range of solutions often works best for most women. So, experiment! You can still have an fulfilling sex life during and after menopause.

SLEEP AND INSOMNIA

Trouble sleeping? Are you waking up at night and having difficulty getting back to sleep? This is yet another common symptom associated with the menopausal transition. And it's a *big* one. Poor sleep spills over into all aspects of our life. It impacts our physical and mental performance, our mood, our alertness levels, and so much more. Interestingly, other symptoms, like hot flashes and anxiety, can lead to a poor sleep. Yet, so can fluctuating hormone levels that impact your circadian rhythm.

Since other symptoms may impact your sleep or contribute to a poor sleep, this is why many women tend to benefit from a combination of treatment approaches when it comes to perimenopause and menopause. Tackling this problem from multiple angles can help ensure you resolve this issue and don't lead the rest of your life in zombie-mode.

CIRCULATION PROBLEMS

Circulation is also affected during menopause. The main culprit is thought to be yet again good ol' estrogen. Of course, other hormones including cortisol and progesterone play a role. In fact, it's really the ratio of all these hormones that gets thrown off during the menopausal transition and leads to various unwanted symptoms.

Furthermore, inflammation may also lead to poor and reduced circulation during menopause. When arteries and veins are affected by inflammation, circulation is reduced, which, in turn, leads to anything from raised blood pressure to swollen or cold feet. Therefore, during menopause, it is essential to keep an eye on your blood pressure. The unfortunate truth is that there is an increased cardiovascular risk during menopause, and we want to limit this (as well as monitor it!) at all costs.

JOINT PAIN DURING MENOPAUSE

There are so many symptoms we don't usually associate with menopause, like joint paint. Joint pain in menopause can cause your neck, knees, shoulders, and really any of your joints to ache. As estrogen levels vary during menopause, so will levels of inflammation in your body, which may affect your joints. Furthermore, when we are mentally or physically stressed, our cortisol levels increase which also leads to joint pain. Talk about feeling old! But again, there's ways to combat and reduce this. So, let's not cycle into ruminating thoughts. Instead, let's move forward and continue to learn why these changes are happening and what we can do about them.

COGNITIVE FUNCTION AND BRAIN FOG

One surprising sign of menopause is brain fog or reduced cognitive function. You may become somewhat forgetful when you used to pride yourself on your recall abilities. You might find yourself foggy and unsure when performing what used to be routine tasks. As ego-crushing as this can be, the good news is that cognitive function does seems to come back. More research is needed to back this up, but the common assumption is that brain fog has to do with those powerful unbalanced hormones, yet again.

Our brain is more reliant on the perfect hormonal balance than we might think. After all, hormones help us sleep. They determine our mood and how we feel. They enhance our alertness or hinder it. They also impact our behavior. With that said, it's a bit of a no-brainer as to why our minds might feel foggy and less-than-optimal during this time. Practice patience and compassion with yourself. It's not you; It's your hormones. In particular, researchers have noted that it's common for menopausal women to have high levels of cortisol. Combine this with fluctuating estrogen levels, and there's going to be misfires and miscommunication within the nervous system. Knowing this is due to the changes that come with menopause can help assure you that there's a temporary reason for it (and that you aren't simply losing your mind!).

YOUR BREASTS AND MENOPAUSE

Increased or new breast pain during menopause comes down almost exclusively to hormonal changes that your body is going through. Interestingly, women who use the contraceptive pill for pregnancy prevention or to control symptoms, experience less breast pain due to better hormonal control. If you experience severe breast pain or discharge from your nipples, it is always best to visit your doctor.

EYESIGHT PROBLEMS IN MENOPAUSE

Our eyesight can deteriorate with age and is also one of the physical effects that you may experience during menopause. This is another symptom doctors don't normally associate with menopause. They often dismiss it as a sign that you are simply getting older.

And while it is not clear whether eyesight problems are *directly* related to menopause, as men often get reading glasses around the same time too, still, you need to be aware that this may be one of the effects on the body that you may experience due to menopause or that may be accelerated because of menopause. So, why might this happen? The reasons are not clear, but it could be that microcirculation to the back of the eyes decreases as a result of changing hormonal levels.

SKIN AND MENOPAUSE

The skin is the body's largest organ. Most of us don't even think of the skin as an organ, but the skin does so much more than just hold us together. It's the first line of defense against foreign invaders. It helps keep us properly hydrated. And it also presents us to the external world. It's no secret that many of us, as we age, concern ourselves with the appearance of our skin as we try to find any answer that allows us to bask in the fountain of youth for just a little bit longer.

During perimenopause, you may notice your skin change. This happens due to declining collagen levels, leading to dullness, reduced elasticity, and wrinkles. Your usual face cream and other skincare products are less likely to be effective at this time. When you notice this, taking a second look at your skincare routine is important. However, that is not the only thing you should do.

It is critical for you to review your diet. Your skin health and appearance is a reflection of what you eat. If you can boost your skin health through your diet and new skincare routines during perimenopause, you will notice your skin will fare better during the actual menopause transition (the year after your last period) and postmenopause.

SKIN ALLERGIES

It is not uncommon to develop allergies and eczema once you enter the menopausal stages of your life. Fortunately, you can combat both naturally and with conventional treatments.

Some women also say they start to experience psoriasis during menopause. Psoriasis is a skin condition where the skin produces excess skin cells and can cause redness and itching. Part of the reason for psoriasis is an increased level of inflammation.

New food allergies may also manifest themselves in the form of a skin allergy or eczema. If you think your rash is a result of a food allergy, keeping a diet or food diary may help. This can determine what may be working within your diet and what might not. Alternatively, you can visit your doctor for an allergy test.

Lastly, if your fashion jewellery starts leading to unpleasant itching (yes, this might happen!), it could mean you have developed a nickel allergy. It is believed that this is caused by increased sensitivity to certain metals during menopause. (Who knew that could be a thing?!)

MENOPAUSE AND HAIR

Don't be surprised if you experience some hair loss or hair thinning during this stage in your life. Again, changes in hormones may lead to thinner hair.

During menopause, your hair may also become dry, resulting in dandruff. However, an easy remedy is dandruff shampoo and hair oils! Massaging the scalp may also improve circulation to this area and enhance the health of the hair follicles, reducing hair thinning and dryness.

CHAPTER FOUR

HOW MENOPAUSE AFFECTS YOUR EMOTIONS & MENTAL HEALTH

"Menopause: It's not just a mood swing, it's a whole damn mood playground."

- Unknown

The mental and emotion turmoil and angst that comes with menopause isn't something to be brushed over. An increase in mental health issues is common during menopause, including depression and anxiety. During this time of life, it's easy to not feel like ourselves. Our bodies have gone rogue and seemingly have a mind of their own. We might feel like we're in a fog or get frustrated and fed up with the rollercoaster of changes and even physical pain we might experience. This is completely understandable. So, let's dig a bit deeper here. What else should you know when it comes to menopause and your emotional and mental health?

ANXIETY AND MENOPAUSE

People experience anxiety for all sorts of reasons. And contrary to popular belief, anxiety goes beyond the simple worries of the day. If we have a particular event coming up, we might feel anxious. If we have to speak in public, we might feel anxious. If we are bothered by a person or situation, we might feel anxious. And during menopause, you might just notice more feelings of anxiety than normal.

You can thank increased cortisol and other fluctuations in our hormones again for this one!

Symptoms of anxiety include:

* Constant worrying

* Trembling and shaking

* Irrational fear

* Repeated flashbacks

* Panic attacks

* Feeling nauseous

* Sadness

* Clammy hands

* New habits such as repeated cleaning and rearranging your environment

Dealing with anxiety is never easy. However, both natural remedies and conventional treatments are available. It is possible to overcome these anxious thoughts and find balance once again.

DEPRESSION AND MENOPAUSE

Feeling a little bit blue or sad is a normal part of life. However, when you feel sad all the time or you feel like you are sinking into a big black hole of despair and hopelessness, the situation is, undeniably, much more serious.

Depression in menopause is very common. It often starts during perimenopause and continues through post menopause then seems to lift when hormones finally balance themselves out and the body gets back to equilibrium.

Symptoms of depression include:

* Low mood for a longer period of time

* Loss of interest in hobbies

* Withdrawing from social activities

* Feelings of fatigue or loss of energy

* Changes in appetite

* Difficulty concentrating and making decisions

* Sleeping too much or too little

* Thoughts of death or suicide

If you have any of the above, don't hesitate to reach out for help. Sometimes, we all need a helping hand.

LOW SELF-ESTEEM

Feeling that your confidence has been knocked down is common during menopause. You may suddenly feel like you can't do the things you used to do, or you lack the confidence to do them. Women often say they experience reduced confidence because their body shape may change during menopause, or they simply don't feel like themselves. Many women gain weight which can be a blow to their wardrobe, ego, and self-esteem.

The truth is that our bodies' appearance often does change in menopause. As we age, our skin starts to wrinkle, and we may put on weight in places where we haven't before. Other parts of our bodies, such as our breasts, may begin to sag and head south for the winter permanently (no matter how much you plead with the girls to stay!).

Experiencing feelings associated with looking less feminine and beautiful is not unusual. And you aren't alone; low confidence and poor self-esteem affect millions of women as they go through their menopausal journeys.

Yet, healthy eating and exercising are fantastic ways to boost your confidence and self-esteem. Exercise, in particular, releases "feel-good" hormones which can work wonders on your mental and emotional well-being. More about this will be discussed later in this book.

CHAPTER FIVE

HOW MENOPAUSE AFFECTS YOUR SEX LIFE

"Menopause: It's like puberty, but in reverse. First you get the hot flashes, then you stop wanting to have sex."

- Unknown

A whole chapter on sex?! Yes, let's go there. A loss of libido (sex drive) during menopause can affect our intimate relationship with our spouse or partner. This can have various negative repercussions on our quality of life. A loss of libido (interest in sex) has its roots in both physical and psychological causes. And a lack of sex drive (much to many women's dismay!) is *very* common in menopause. Not only does the female body produce the female hormone, estrogen, but it also produces testosterone which is the male hormone. However, the rate at which testosterone is produced declines during menopause, giving way to less interest in getting down and dirty.

In fact, testosterone levels fall naturally in both men and women with age; it is not only women who experience lower levels. In women, testosterone levels vary all the time. Menopause plays a role in this, but there are other times when women's testosterone level falls. Good examples are after childbirth and surgery.

Stress, depression, and anxiety also affect the libido. Conventional medications for depression and anxiety, may make you feel happier but, they can actually further lower your libido and make you feel less sexy—a trade-off you definitely want to take into consideration before diving headfirst. Hormone replacement and the use of hormone-based contraception are other possibilities to consider (more on this coming up!).

CONVENTIONAL TREATMENTS FOR LOW LIBIDO

So, how can you get your (in the words of Justin Timberlake) "sexy back"? Conventional treatments for low libido may include testosterone implants or injections. Testosterone treatments may also help with other health problems you experience during menopause, including poor sleep and loss of muscle tone.

SELF-HELP

Many women seem to prefer self-help treatments when it comes to the loss of libido. Popular options are herbal remedies or just general self-care that may work wonders on boosting your self-esteem, such as going for beauty treatments and massages which can help you relax. After all, a big part of getting down and dirty involves getting out of your own head and learning to enjoy the moment.

THE MIND AND LIBIDO

As hinted above, there is a mind and body connection in relation to the libido. Women often say that a range of complementary therapies has helped them regain their libido, including stress-reducing techniques and more. If we think of libido as a kind of energy, it may make it easier to understand.

Perhaps, during this time, energy is simply redirected to other vital functions. From a psychological point of view, you can say that energy may be directed to other activities women see as more important. After all, as we can't have children after menopause, it could be considered somewhat natural that our energy be focused somewhere else. Of course, when you're in a relationship, there is another person involved and your loss of libido may have a big impact on your relationship and intimacy. After all, sex fosters connection and feelings of closeness for many people. It's also a source of pleasure for you and your partner to enjoy together. On top of this, regular sex has many health benefits like reduced stress, enhanced sleep, and even better immunity. All of this is to say is that there's more to losing one's libido than *simply* sex. And there's various reasons you may want to ignite that spark once again and seek out ways to improve your sex drive—all of which are completely understandable and justified. So, all the power to you! If you want to regain your sex drive, you *can* and you *will*. It all comes down to exploring what works for you and your life. So, let's take a look at a few alternative ways you can reclaim your sexual self!

ALTERNATIVE WAYS TO REGAIN LIBIDO

Aromatherapy

Essential oils can help to alleviate feelings of tension and stress. Jasmine is one oil that is well-known for its libido-enhancing qualities. Another popular oil is ylang-ylang.

Rosemary oil on the other hand is a fantastic oil for increasing blood circulation which influences vaginal dryness and indirectly, libido. Consider sensual massages with your partner or a little self-care routine with these oils before getting in between the sheets. Maybe it's just what you need to feel that fire once again.

Nutritional therapy

There are also various foods that can help you to boost your libido. We know that foods rich in potassium are excellent for our libido. Oysters are considered good source of potassium, perhaps that's why they are often referred to as an aphrodisiac. Some common, everyday foods are further packed with potassium, including bananas, avocados, oats, broccoli, and potatoes.

Believe it or not, eating smaller and lighter meals may also help you on your libido crusade. As we age, the body finds it harder to generate energy from food. When you eat smaller and lighter meals, the body starts to make the most of what you eat, without overburdening the digestive system.

One quick thing to note is that sugar lowers your libido. If you eat a lot of sugary snacks or foods (particularly processed or pre-packaged food items full of *refined* sugar) that are converted into sugar in the body, you may find yourself experiencing a lower libido. Hence, in order to improve your libido, you may want to take your diet into serious consideration.

Energy healing systems

Many energy healing and balancing systems, such as yoga and tai-chi, may also aid in boosting your sex drive.

Acupuncture and Traditional Chinese Medicine ("TCM"), as discussed later in this book, have a long history of helping when it comes to energy healing. The way TCM is used differs vastly from Western medicine. Many practices within TCM including herbalism and cupping can have positive effects on more than just your libido. In other words, they won't just help you rediscover your sexy side but also enhance your overall health and well-being.

CHAPTER SIX

HORMONES AND MENOPAUSE

"At her first bleeding, a woman meets her power. During her bleeding years, she practices it. At menopause, she becomes it."

- Traditional Native American saying

HRT is one hot topic. Should you or shouldn't you? The debate continues and it is often a heated one. To better understand HRT and women's health, you need to know how HRT treatments work. They can have positive effects as well as negative effects. External factors also play a role on how your body responds to HRT. As previously mentioned, hormones are often added to animal feed. They work their way down the food chain ending up in the food we eat. There is a possibility that this hormonal residue may influence how you respond to HRT.

Over the years, HRT has received a lot of negative publicity which has caused fear and uncertainty about taking it. However, it is vital to note that we all react differently when it comes to medical treatments. If you decide that HRT is right for you, work together with your doctor to find the best one specific for you.

Currently, HRT treatments are available as tablets, creams, suppositories, skin patches, and implants. This is a very fast-moving field of medicine, so new ways of delivering HRT are emerging all the time. HRT can actually be quite useful for many women, when implemented and used at the right time and for the right purpose. For instance, recent research shows that HRT is better implemented early and *before* menopause (within 5-10 years of menopause) to support health and vitality, including potentially reducing the risk of cardiovascular disease and enhancing bone health. When implemented *after* menopause, it can actually have detrimental effects on health. So, let's expand our knowledge on this topic a bit more.

KEY HORMONES AFFECTED BY MENOPAUSE

The three primary hormones affected by menopause are estrogen, progesterone, and testosterone. However, those are not the only hormones affected by menopause. As there is an imbalance between the three primary hormones, other hormones are affected as well. One follows the other and the overall lowering or imbalance of certain hormones may have a domino effect on our entire well-being.

To truly understand how Hormone Replacement Therapy ("HRT") works, you need to be aware that the levels of cortisol, serotonin, dopamine, and melatonin are also impacted. When you take estrogen, you improve the overall hormonal balance in the body. This is why HRT can be so effective when it comes to women's health. Now, let's take a closer look at these hormones to get a clearer picture of HRT.

ESTROGEN

Both men and women have the hormone, estrogen, in their bodies but women create more of it. The ovaries, adrenal glands, and fat tissues produce estrogen. It not only makes us feminine, but it controls the menstrual cycle and is also "responsible" for the urinary tract, breasts, and mucus membranes. It also plays a vital role when it comes to the heart and cardiovascular system. A lack of estrogen can cause the arteries to become inflamed which can lead to a narrowing of the arterial walls. As estrogen continues to decline as we go through menopause, we are more likely to experience heart disease, as mentioned previously in this book.

When estrogen levels drop, we are also more likely to experience problems with our bones which can lead to osteoporosis. We develop wrinkles and can experience problems with our hair. A low level of estrogen leads to weaker pelvic muscles. Furthermore, the reason many women feel they experience depression or reduced cognitive function is because of lower estrogen levels in the brain. At the end of the day, estrogen does much more than regulate the menstrual cycle.

PROGESTERONE

Although it is the progesterone's job to get the uterus ready for pregnancy, it has other important functions in the body. Just like estrogen, it is a female sex hormone. A 2003 study mentioned on the leading clinical website NCBI showed that progesterone helps to protect against ovarian cancer. In recent years, we have started to learn more about progesterone and have found that it may be linked to the sleep cycle. One thing we do know is that falling progesterone levels in menopause, coupled with an increase in the production of the hormone cortisol, leads to weight gain. This explains why many women gain weight during menopause. Progesterone further has a calming effect, which means when levels fluctuate, anxiety is also common.

TESTOSTERONE

Many women think of testosterone as only a male hormone but the ovaries and the adrenal glands in women also produce testosterone. Normal levels of testosterone in women help to regulate our mood and sleep. However, that's not all.

Testosterone also has physical functions; it supports the skeletal and reproductive systems. On top of that, it helps us build muscle and promotes healthy hair growth. As the ovaries start to shut down, the level of testosterone declines rather quickly. For instance, you may notice far less hair growth on your legs as well as a loss in muscle tone.

CORTISOL

Often dubbed the "stress hormone," cortisol is known as a steroid hormone. It is produced by your adrenal glands which are located on top of the kidneys.

It is the job of cortisol to regulate our body's response to stress. Cortisol also stimulates fat and carbohydrate metabolism (It's not just about stress here!). In menopause, when all the hormones go haywire, cortisol is also impacted. Thus, it's harder to control stress and subsequently, metabolism. As estrogen falls, cortisol takes over some of its functions including inflammation suppression and blood sugar regulation.

Cortisol's ultimate goal in the body is to help the body achieve homeostasis (all systems functioning equally and at optimum levels). However, with so much going on internally during menopause, there is little wonder that it falls short. It puts digestion on the back burner which is why women in menopause may experience excess tummy fat and gastrointestinal distress or changes. Scientists aren't entirely sure, but they think cortisol may interpret menopause as a time of chronic stress. In turn, this can cause a handful of issues.

Cortisol also affects your sleep cycle. To help cortisol balance and work toward homeostasis, we can reduce stress through various strategies and practices (like meditation, yoga, deep breathing, etc.) and adequate exercise. Weight training and increasing muscle mass seems to be particularly helpful. Yet, as per usual, more research is needed to find out the importance of cortisol in menopause.

SEROTONIN

Serotonin is a neurotransmitter that acts as a hormone. It is a powerful chemical that helps control your wellbeing and happiness. If you are not getting enough of it, you may experience irritability, anxiety, and depression. When our bodies produce a good level of serotonin, we sleep better and feel happier.

Interestingly, the hormones that oversee your menstrual cycle also help manage and regulate serotonin. Thus, when these hormones fluctuate or fall, we experience fluctuations and declines in serotonin (and our mood!). Since the gut actually produces about 95% of the body's serotonin, these changes may also be attributed to inflammation or issues with digestion. Fix your gut, and you might just fix most of your serotonin issues.

DOPAMINE

Dopamine is both a hormone and a neurotransmitter. Many doctors like to call it the "happiness hormone" as it makes its' function in the body easier to understand. Dopamine can indeed help to make us feel happy, but there is more to dopamine than happiness.

Dopamine helps to support memory, movement and most importantly, motivation. During menopause, a woman's dopamine levels decrease. This may be the reason why menopausal women say they feel flat or unmotivated. Although, more studies are needed, it is believed that the drop in estrogen and progesterone levels, reduce dopamine levels and may increase inflammation in parts of the brain.

As many women in menopause mention problems with memory and cognitive function, there is every possibility that there is a link between dopamine and memory loss during menopause. Although, yet again, more research is needed to clarify and identify if there is a specific link to women in menopause (C'mon, science, catch up!).

MELATONIN

Melatonin is a hormone produced in the brain that helps control the release of female reproductive hormones. As estrogen levels fall, melatonin production appears to struggle with self-regulation. This can lead to symptoms of fatigue, exhaustion, and insomnia.

A 2014 Finnish study by Elan Toffol MD of 250 menopausal women suggests that melatonin may be the culprit behind intense night sweats and hot flashes. Over a three-month period, 250 women, ages 43 to 71 years of age, were asked to take a melatonin supplement every day. This helped reduce both hot flashes and night sweats, giving them a night of better sleep. When these women woke up in the morning, they found that they had slept better and had more energy.

Aging, in general, influences melatonin production in the body. According to a study carried out in 2017 and published in NCBI, there is a link between menopause, sleep, and hot flashes. If the circadian rhythm (our sleep-wake cycle) is disturbed when melatonin levels decrease, there is a possibility that this can also lead to vasomotor problems and arrhythmias (an irregular heartbeat). Complicated, I know. But our hormones truly are worth understanding, especially since they are the ones going a bit haywire during menopause.

CHAPTER SEVEN

HORMONE REPLACEMENT THERAPY (HRT)

"Hormones are the chemical messengers that allow our bodies to communicate with each other and keep everything working together in harmony."

- Unknown

HRT is a conventional treatment for many menopausal issues and symptoms. If you do decide to use HRT to reduce your menopausal symptoms, it's important to feel confident in your decision. Sadly, doctors are not always good at explaining treatment choices (nor do many of them have much time as they try to see as many people as possible during their busy schedules). On top of this, there are tons of myths and misconceptions when it comes to HRT. This is why we're going into a bit more detail in this book. Let's find out what exactly HRT is all about and determine whether it is or may eventually be the right option for you.

HRT comes in many shapes and sizes! Today, you can choose between tablets, creams, suppositories, and skin patches. The Mirena IUD is an implant you may want to consider during perimenopause and there is even a spray

HRT. In the future, we are likely to see more HRT sprays and maybe even other options.

There are no hard or fast rules when choosing HRT. More so, it is often a game of trial and error. When it comes to choosing an HRT option (or forgoing it altogether!), decide what is best for you, your personal circumstances, and your needs. Remember, every woman is different. Just because Julie down the street uses HRT or a certain type of HRT, it doesn't necessarily mean it's right for you. So, let's dig a little deeper, shall we?

HRT PILLS

Many of the studies we read about HRT involve pills or tablets. Combined estrogen and progesterone pills are the most popular option if you haven't had a period for over 15 months. During perimenopause, you may want to try out sequential combined HRT. This is a treatment containing a daily dose of estrogen with a variable amount of progesterone in each cycle. As the hormone supply is varied, it means you may experience a bleed every month or every couple of months.

New HRT pill brands tend to hit the market on a fairly regular basis, but some brands have stood the test of time. And interestingly, the hormonal components of the brands are very similar; however, your doctor may have a preference or there could be a slight variation in price, ultimately, making the decision for you.

If you have had a hysterectomy and don't need progesterone, you will probably be recommended an estrogen-only HRT tablet.

So, a big question you might have… can you take HRT pills if you are already receiving estrogen spray or gel? If you are concerned about oral estrogen and use another delivery method, surprisingly, you may still benefit from taking oral progesterone.

Another quick note here: Some hormone tablets contain estrogens derived from horses. If you don't want to take these kinds of tablets for ethical or any other reasons, you should mention this to your doctor.

THE BENEFITS OF HRT PILLS

Taking a pill or tablet is convenient; you can easily add it to your daily routine. If you are already taking medication for something else, taking an HRT pill may fit easily into your already existing routine.

Many women like to take pills as they don't have to worry about skin contact. With the patch, some women may discover an allergy to the fabric in the patch. The hormones can also cause skin irritations. That is why you need to place them on different parts of the body, and this is definitely something you want to be aware of before making any one decision.

THE DOWNSIDES TO HRT PILLS

With HRT pills, there is a slightly increased risk of Deep Vein Thrombosis or a pulmonary embolism, but the risk is very low. If you have a family history of circulatory disease or thrombosis, it is important to be aware of this history to avoid the use of the HRT pills which may result in blood clots.

Some women say they find it hard to remember to take HRT pills during menopause. If you struggle with remembering to take tablets, you can buy a day-of-the-week pillbox or opt for patches instead.

HRT PATCHES

Many women use HRT patches which, basically, look like a band-aid. These patches can be adhered to your skin and are a convenient way of delivering HRT as your patch will last between three to four days. Easy!

BENEFITS OF USING HRT PATCHES

It is believed that HRT patches reduce the risk of blood clots. As the hormones in patches are directly released into the bloodstream, they bypass the liver, which may decrease this risk. However, it is worth emphasizing that it is only a consideration. Additionally, women often claim they experience fewer side effects, such as nausea and headaches, when they use patches. Thus, for some, the patch reigns supreme!

THE DOWNSIDES TO HRT PATCHES

What goes up must come down. HRT patches, inevitably, have their downsides, such as skin irritations. If you have sensitive skin or a pre-existing skin condition, you may want to avoid patches. Also, if you swim or sweat a lot, the absorption rate of hormones may be slightly erratic (meaning its effects could be somewhat inconsistent).

When you use patches, you may also experience indigestion and bloating, despite not taking the hormones orally. You may also experience more weight fluctuations with patches. However, side effects always depend on the person and may vary (or even not occur at all).

HRT GELS

HRT gels are becoming more and more popular. These gels contain estrogen, which you spread onto the skin. Using the skin as the delivery system, HRT gels get directly absorbed into the bloodstream. The best places to apply HRT gels are on the inner thigh or outer arm. The best time to apply them is generally considered to be after a shower. Then, you need to give them a minimum of five minutes to dry naturally.

Once you have applied the gel, you should not use any skincare treatments or body lotions for at least one hour. And you won't want to apply it before a workout or swim as perspiration and water make gels less effective.

What you also need to know is that there is a difference between vaginal and topical gels. You can't use a vaginal gel on your skin and vice versa.

THE BENEFITS OF HRT GELS

Just like patches, gels reduce the risk of blood clots. One of the main benefits of gels is that the dosage is easier to adjust. Many women say they easily find the right "level" to control their menopausal symptoms when using gels.

Thankfully, you do not need to worry about applying the wrong dosage because HRT gels are packaged in pumps that deliver the correct dosage for you. The dose is something you discuss with your doctor. The most common dose is one or two "pumps."

THE DOWNSIDES OF HRT GELS

Some think that these gels are sticky and take a long time to dry. While you do need to allow time for the gel to dry, many women don't find this too inconvenient. Yet, this may come down to your specific lifestyle and is something to consider.

If you still have a uterus (aka you haven't had a hysterectomy), you need to take progesterone alongside HRT gels. Although, there are bioidentical progesterone gels and creams, they have not been tested for effectiveness yet (To be continued!).

HRT SPRAYS

An increasing number of medical treatments are delivered using sprays. We already use spray-type treatments for hay fever and allergies. At the end of the day, sprays are effective and convenient ways of delivering a medication directly into the bloodstream. At the time of writing this, there is only one HRT spray available in the US. In the future, we are likely to see more HRT sprays (Remember, this is an ever-growing field of research with a growing market!).

THE BENEFITS OF HRT SPRAYS

As each spray only contains a measured amount of HRT, there is no way (or almost no way besides getting the number of sprays wrong) you can take too much. Once again, it is thought that the risk of experiencing blood clots is reduced when taking HRT sprays.

Just like a perfume, you can take your spray with you everywhere you go, which makes it easy to use at any time. You don't have to worry about skin irritations, as in the case of using patches. Unlike gels, you don't have to wait for the gel to dry. Lots of upsides here for the modern woman!

THE DOWNSIDES OF HRT SPRAYS

Even though a spray is convenient, you still need to remember to administer it. It's further preferable to use the spray at the same time every day, which can be tedious for some to keep up with.

Furthermore, do not fall into the trap that the more sprays you use, the better. To avoid hormonal imbalances, you should always stick to the agreed dosage (which is a number of sprays as per your doctor's instructions).

VAGINAL HRT

If you are experiencing burning, itching and tightness in your vagina, then you may be a candidate for vaginal HRT. Other symptoms that may require the use of this treatment include painful sex and frequent urination. Your doctor will call your symptoms genitourinary or GSM for short. You may also hear the terms atrophic vaginitis or vaginal atrophy. This, unfortunately, means the vagina is thinning, becoming dry, or becoming inflamed. While this may sound embarrassing, it's a very common issue for many menopausal women and it can be addressed through HRT (No shame, ladies!).

Specifically, if these are your only symptoms during menopause, they are easily treated with vaginal HRT. This kind of treatment involves the application of estrogen directly to the vaginal area. Pessaries and vaginal tablets are okay, however, if you suffer from vaginal atrophy, you may find them challenging to insert. Vaginal gels have many of the same attributes as creams and you can use them the same way. So, let's take a closer look at this type of HRT. How can you keep "down there" in better shape with HRT throughout your menopausal journey?

THE BENEFITS OF VAGINAL HRT

Vaginal HRT is often referred to as the most "risk-free" HRT. From what we know, there are no links to blood clots, cancer, or stroke when you use vaginal HRT. The potential reason for this is that the hormones are directly applied to the affected area. This means they don't go through the bloodstream or act on any other organs or system within the body (at least, so the theory goes).

THE DOWNSIDES OF VAGINAL HRT

The major downside to this treatment is that vaginal HRT is only going to help you manage localized symptoms in your vagina. If you are experiencing other symptoms, such as hot flashes and mood changes, vaginal HRT is not going to help and you may need other remedies or strategies to aid your menopausal transition.

VAGINAL RINGS

A vaginal ring is a rather new way of delivering localized HRT. In this treatment method, a ring is inserted into the vagina. Over time, the soft ring gradually releases estrogen making your genitourinary track health that much better. The ring needs to be changed every three months.

THE MIRENA IUD

The primary function of the Mirena IUD is to prevent pregnancy. However, recently, doctors have started to use it as a form of "early HRT." If you are experiencing perimenopause symptoms with heavy bleeding, the Mirena IUD may be a good option. It sits securely in the womb releasing progesterone at a continuous rate which prevents the uterus from thickening and thus, results in lighter (and potentially less painful) periods.

THE BENEFITS OF THE MIRENA IUD

With the Mirena IUD, you get two benefits. First, it prevents pregnancy which can still happen during perimenopause and second, it reduces bleeding. In addition, it lasts for 4-5 years so once it is inserted you don't have to worry about birth control and you should have lighter periods. You also won't have to remember to take a pill or replace your patch (all wins!).

When experiencing other symptoms, you should discuss what other options you can use with your Mirena IUD. An estrogen spray, patch, or tablet may be used in tandem with the Mirena IUD to help with other symptoms. As always, it's best to bring this up with your doctor as they know you and your health situation that best and can help you navigate the appropriate option for you.

THE DOWNSIDES OF THE MIRENA IUD

Depending on your health insurance, the Mirena IUD has a higher upfront cost and needs to be inserted by an OB-GYN doctor.

The first couple of weeks can be uncomfortable as your body adjusts to the IUD. You may experience bleeding, cramps, and pinching. However, as the body gets used to the IUD, most women say that they feel much better and experience various benefits (as mentioned above).

CHAPTER EIGHT

GETTING STARTED WITH HRT

"Medicine is a science of uncertainty and an art of probability."
- William Osler

While there are drug stores out there that will probably allow you to buy HRT without a prescription, it's best not to self-medicate. A range of health considerations need to be considered. With so many treatments available, it's not always easy or as straightforward process to find the right one that suits your needs.

Sometimes, you may need to try different forms and brands of HRT before you find the right one. For instance, one brand of HRT may cause breakthrough bleeds while another will not. And again, this varies from woman to woman. Your family doctor or OB-GYN can help to point you in the right direction here.

Don't be afraid to discuss treatments or bring up your concerns with your doctor. When you start considering HRT, discussing the options available is important. Patches are easy to use and so are pills. Creams can be hard to measure out and suppositories can be messy. When you choose an implant, removing it may be challenging. Hence, you must discuss this with your doctor and find one or a combination that suits your body and lifestyle.

You need to have confidence in your choice of HRT. If your doctor does not create an environment where you can talk about what choices are available, it might be time to find another doctor (I'm serious!). Awareness is one of the most important parts of HRT. And just like any other profession, there are good doctors and not so good doctors. Find yourself a good one that takes the time to discuss the options rather than one that simply throws a band-aid solution on the problem or concerns you bring up.

WHEN TO START HRT

Not all women start taking HRT post menopause. In fact, there is some evidence showing it may be *more* beneficial to take HRT before menopause. Thus, many women start taking HRT during perimenopause. It all depends on your circumstances and how you are feeling; you need to be honest with yourself and your doctor. Before you visit a doctor, it is a good idea to write down all of your signs and symptoms; this will make your doctor's job easier and help both of you have an informed discussion. Don't be surprised if your doctor recommends the contraceptive pill instead when you go to him or her with your signs and symptoms. It has been shown that some contraceptive pills can have a positive effect during perimenopause.

One thing that the contraceptive pill is very good at during perimenopause is to help regulate periods and manage weight.

Deciding when you should start taking HRT is not an easy choice. Never be afraid to ask questions and don't feel embarrassed about it.

CHECK-UP DURING HRT

Most healthy women don't have a problem when taking HRT, but just in case, your doctor will probably do a couple of basic health checks. You may have to take a blood test to measure your hormone and cholesterol levels. Your doctor may also take your blood pressure, listen to your heart, and check your weight. Your doctor may also ask about your family health history. A history of heart issues and/ or breast cancer will affect the type of HRT prescribed.

The thing is hormones are tricky. They impact the body in more ways than one. I could go on for a whole book (or more) about HRT and the hormones involved, as well as their impacts on the body. But I imagine no one would read that book so this whole section is about handing off what you *need* to know. If you're curious beyond what's in the pages of this book, I encourage you to do your own research. Getting thoroughly informed and finding the answers to your questions can help guide your decision-making process and your menopausal *and* health journey.

SIGNS THAT SHOW YOU NEED HRT

One of the first signs that you've entered perimenopause is often irregular periods. Your periods may come closer to each other and may be heavier or lighter. Some women end up with periods lasting for several weeks before they get a short break. It is important to monitor erratic and heavy periods as they often lead to anemia. In cases where severe changes have occurred, such as increased pain or heavy bleeding, HRT may be appropriate.

Other symptoms to look out for when considering if HRT is right for you include night sweats, mood swings, sleep issues, hot flashes, hair loss, and urinary tract problems. HRT is often considered when symptoms are severe or begin to drastically impact a woman's everyday life. On top of these symptoms, you may find yourself experiencing vaginal itching, burning, and dryness. Again, if these become disruptive, HRT may pose a viable option. (Let's be honest: None of us want an itchy vagina distracting us during that social event or big work project!)

THE FIRST MONTH OF HRT TREATMENT

During the first month of taking HRT, you may notice breast tenderness, bloating, and/or some bleeding as your body adjusts to the hormones. On a positive note, you may also notice better sleep and higher energy levels which should make you feel better and improve your mood.

Everybody is different so it is important to keep a log or notebook. You never quite know what is happening unless it's tracked! At the end of every month, create a list of the benefits and any negative side-effects you may be experiencing. Alternatively, you may want to track your mood, symptoms, and more each day to keep a firm accountability on what is happening with you and your body. This can also serve as a list of concerns or questions to bring up with your doctor at your next appointment.

HRT AND SIDE EFFECTS

As you probably already gathered from previous sections in this book, side effects with HRT are entirely possible. The most common side effects of HRT are headaches, nausea, and breast pain, as well as indigestion and even leg cramps. As side effects vary so much from one woman to the next, it is important to be aware of what to expect. If your HRT does not contain progesterone, you may also experience bloating. Vaginal bleeding is further a common side-effect that you need to discuss with your doctor. While it may not be dangerous, vaginal bleeding is the one thing most women on HRT would rather not have. After all, this big transition is usually about less bleeding (with the eventual halting of your menstrual cycle altogether), not more!

STATINS AND HRT

With rising obesity levels and heart disease, statins are a popular medication used to lower cholesterol. It is not clear whether taking a statin and HRT together has negative side effects. However, there is some evidence from Scandinavian studies that seems to indicate that the two don't work well together. If you are taking statins as well as HRT, you may experience increased side effects when compared to the norm. These may include headaches, nausea, vertigo, and dizziness. You should also look out for tiredness and muscle pain. If you experience any of these, make sure to talk to your doctor as soon as you can.

HYSTERECTOMY AND MENOPAUSE

During a hysterectomy, most doctors remove both the ovaries and the uterus. There are occasions when the surgeon does not remove the ovaries. If your ovaries are not removed, you shouldn't experience any symptoms related to rapid-onset menopause. Once your uterus and/or ovaries have been removed, you will not need HRT treatment that includes progesterone. Additionally, doctors often like to wait to see how a woman's body has responded to the hysterectomy before introducing any hormones or other strategies.

If you had a complete hysterectomy, you may experience a rapid onset of menopause. Some women say they experience symptoms straight away or within a matter of days. The truth is that experiences vary a great deal. If you are a woman who has been through menopause before your hysterectomy, you should not "technically" experience a return of symptoms or new symptoms. Nevertheless, many women say that they do.

Women who have been through a hysterectomy often say they experience more intense breast pain. The reason for that is not clearly understood yet. But, as always, it's likely related to hormonal levels fluctuating quite drastically.

Another common symptom that you may experience post-hysterectomy is headaches. Yet, when it comes to hot flashes, it normally takes some time for you to experience them. What matters is to be open-minded and take each day as it comes after a hysterectomy. One of the best things you can do is to write down of symptoms. When you go for a check-up, talk them through with your doctor.

And here's another quick truth: hormonal imbalances may take time to make themselves known; your diet and lifestyle are major influencing factors. Tracking your symptoms and discussing them with your doctor is important. It helps you and educates your doctor, helping you both get a grip on the whole picture. In turn, this can lead to a more informed discussion and treatment or management strategy.

HRT STUDIES

In the early 2000s, a couple of very slanted studies were produced which would seem to indicate that there is an increased risk of breast cancer and other forms of cancer when HRT therapy was used during menopause and postmenopause. In 2019, an article was published in the British Medical Journal. It was a meta-analysis, which means the analysis took into account many other studies that had been carried out previously.

According to this analysis, there was a greater chance of developing breast cancer if they used HRT for an extended period of time. The risk of developing breast cancer after 10 years of using HRT was said to be doubled. Women who used HRT for a period of 5 years had a lower risk of developing breast cancer. Dr Robert Langer, a member of the board of the International Menopause Society, was quick to point out that the risks were overstated (Not a huge shocker! This isn't the first-time previous studies have led the public astray). The science in the original studies which made up the meta-analysis was not applicable to modern HRT regimes. Dr Robert Langer stressed that HRT helps to protect women from other serious illnesses associated with menopause including cardiovascular diseases and osteoporosis (contrary to popular belief!).

The International Menopause Society also pointed out that data needed to be viewed with caution because of another significant reason; it was not clear how many women who went through menopause early, before the age of 45, would have gone on to develop breast cancer.

While it is important to acknowledge that negative studies are "out there," it is equally important to acknowledge that there were some major problems with these studies. The HRT regimens used in the studies were not indicated. As we have learned more on HRT treatments, the composition of HRT treatments has changed. In general, it is considered that HRT has more positive benefits than serious negative side effects.

There is also another study that is often referred to when it comes to HRT called WHI, or the Women's Health Initiative. The study was published in 1999 but has now come under severe criticism. The main reason for the criticism is the age group that was studied. The average age of the women in that study was 62.7 years. Also, many women in the study were already experiencing a range of health conditions including cardiovascular disease and cerebral problems. Today, if the same study was carried out, we would see greater inclusion of women in a younger age group, that is, between 43 to 55 years. As we age, our immune systems may become compromised and develop cancer for other reasons. Just like we can't blame sugar solely for the obesity epidemic (FYI calories and other factors play a huge role as well), these issues can't be solely attributed to HRT.

Since then, we have learned a lot more and, thankfully, doctors are more aware than in the past. As with any medical therapy or treatment, there are concerns, but we need to look at the background information and the details. For instance, did any of these women have a genetic link to breast cancer? The way we consider and handle clinical evidence has changed vastly since the early 2000s. When studies are carried out now, science and medical technology allow us to take many other factors into account (and prevent us non-scientific folk from being led astray when it comes to our health and medical decisions).

HRT has many health benefits when it comes to women's health. The more we discover about it, the more we start to appreciate that it saves many women's lives, specifically thanks to a lower incidence of heart attacks and other serious health conditions that can start in menopause. On top of that, it probably helps relationships and keeps both men and women sane during a challenging time in a woman's life. And as many of us know, it's our relationships that make this crazy thing called life truly meaningful.

CHAPTER NINE

ALTERNATIVE THERAPIES IN MENOPAUSE

"The greatest medicine of all is to teach people how not to need it."
– Hippocrates

When it comes to women's health, both complementary and alternative medicine have played a huge role. Not all women react well to conventional and Western medicine. Hence, many women are keen on trying out alternative health solutions. If you have had a negative reaction to conventional HRT, you may want to discuss the alternatives with your physician. And fortunately, we live in a time where there are plenty of alternatives to hormone-based replacement. You aren't confined to synthetic hormones, ladies!

So, in this section, we are looking at complementary and alternative health solutions to menopause. What is out there? What might help you through this turbulent transitional time?

WHAT IS COMPLEMENTARY MEDICINE?

Complementary and conventional medicine adopt different approaches when it comes to the definition and treatment of disease. Conventional medicine is diagnosis-led. Doctors use medical tests and symptoms to assess the problem, then treatment is prescribed accordingly.

Many argue that this is a "band-aid" approach that may not always resolve problems but, instead, merely disguises the symptoms.

Complementary practitioners, on the other hand, look at their patients in a holistic manner, meaning they treat the whole person, both physically and mentally, and don't just focus on symptoms *only*. According to complementary medicine principles, illness or health problems signify a disruption of physical and mental well-being. Treatment in complementary medicine focuses on the body's natural self-healing and regulatory abilities. In many ways, it aligns with the body's natural processes. So, what options are there for menopausal women in the complementary medicine realm?

ALTERNATIVE THERAPY

When it comes to alternative therapies in menopause, there are no hard or fast rules. The truth? As always, it tends to depend on each person. Everybody is different. Thus, the combination of therapies that work for you may not always work for others and vice versa.

Below is a list of the alternative and complementary therapies that may be of help during menopause.

* Massage

* Aromatherapy

* Acupuncture

* Yoga

* Naturopathy

* Homeopathy

* Western herbalism

* Chinese Herbalism

* Nutritional Therapies

* Psychotherapy and counselling

* Meditation

* Visualization

We will not go into details of all these suggested complementary therapies however it is good for you to know that they are available. Seek them out in your local area if you want to give them a try and do some self-experimenting. We are instead going to discuss the following alternative therapies in greater detail: Chinese herbalism acupuncture, aromatherapy, homeopathy, naturopathy, and Western herbalism.

It is important to note that there is no real difference between alternative and complementary therapies. Most people believe they fit under the same umbrella, yet medical practitioners believe that there is a slight difference.

Alternative therapies often mean not using any conventional treatments at all. Complementary therapies indicate that therapies may go hand in hand with conventional medicine. Again, the one you choose to go with, very much depends on you.

If you are using conventional HRT, you may experience side effects. When you are being treated for menopause by a doctor, it is important that you discuss any alternatives that you are thinking about trying. It is important if you are thinking about adding herbal supplements to your daily routine when using conventional HRT. Why?

Well, complimentary or alternative therapies may have negative side effects just like conventional therapies do. Some may even contra-indicate. For instance, a qualified homeopath knows never to give the homeopathy remedy, Sepia, to someone using HRT or hormone-based contraception. While many other homeopathy treatments are perfectly safe when used in combination with hormone therapies, Sepia is not. It is a bit like antibiotics and HRT; they should not be used together. Both Sepia and antibiotics disrupt the endocrine system, rendering HRT useless.

So does St John's Wort, which is used as a remedy for depression. It shouldn't be used together with conventional treatments for depression and anxiety. Before combining any therapies, it's essential that you check with your doctor or practitioner as to whether it's safe or not.

CHAPTER TEN

CHINESE HERBALISM

"In Chinese medicine, herbs are not seen as a magic cure-all, but rather as a tool to help the body restore balance and harmony."

– Li Dongyuan

Traditional Chinese Medicine (TCM) is an ancient system of healing dating back thousands of years ago. It has its foundation in the individual diagnosis of symptoms rather than naming a specific disease or health condition.

Chinese herbalism is only one element of TCM. Herbal remedies and dietary regimes are also part of TCM. The basic concepts of energy healing and yin/yang are hard to grasp when you're used to Western medicine. One main concerns of Chinese herbalism is the side effects of some of the ingredients found in Chinese herbs. However, knowledge is power! And standing the test of time, these Chinese remedies definitely have their place.

THE THEORY BEHIND CHINESE MEDICINE

Chinese medicine views health issues as disharmony within the body. In other words, the yin and yang forces in the body are out of balance. TCM also has a principle of following the five elements which are fire, wood, water, metal, and earth. This is a very different viewpoint as far as Western doctors are concerned. And for some, they may even brush it off as a little "woo-woo." Yet, various research and studies have shown its' benefits and uses, despite potentially not entirely knowing how these remedies work within the body.

HOW CHINESE HERBS CAN BENEFIT YOU IN MENOPAUSE

There are a few Chinese herbs that are well-documented for having a positive effect on menopause. For instance, some forms of ginseng and the herb, Dong Quai, are thought to have positive effects. Very little research has been carried out on Dong Quai, but it is believed to contain isoflavones, which are thought to exhibit anti-inflammatory, antioxidant, and antimicrobial properties. Hence, why it might help with certain menopausal symptoms!

It is important to reiterate that each person, in TCM, is seen as an individual. Different herbs and therapies are used for different individuals based on their individual needs and responses. This is what makes Chinese Herbalism difficult to completely figure out and understand. For instance, tea therapies may be recommended. Certain exercises and relaxation techniques have also proven to be useful. But, again, it depends.

EVIDENCE AND RESEARCH

Extensive research into the Chinese herbal side of TCM has been carried out in China. The problem is that formulas used in Chinese herbalism are individually adjusted. It is not believed that one size fits all. Hence, finding enough evidence to prove that TCM works is challenging. Although, there is some evidence and the fact that it's been around for so long is something to be said.

MEDICAL OPINION

In recent years, interest has grown when it comes to Chinese herbalism, particularly outside of China and Asia. Western medicine practitioners are slowly beginning to realize that personal prescriptions and individual dosages may be the way of the future (Finally! We've been shouting about our uniqueness for decades).

ANOTHER SIDE OF TCM: THE INS AND OUTS OF ACUPUNCTURE

Another aspect of TCM is Acupuncture. With acupuncture, practitioners use fine sterile needles that are inserted into specific points of the body. In the West, acupuncture gained steam during the 1970s due to extensive press coverage. Around this time, many Western doctors started using it when all else had failed. To their surprise, it often helped to improve a patient's condition and health outcomes. Acupuncture seems to have a positive effect on the body's energy level specifically, with many claiming they experience a boost of energy after a session.

If you try acupuncture, expect your first acupuncture session to be rather long. The first part will consist of a consultation and then a diagnosis. Normally, no other diagnostic tools are used besides visual diagnosis and pulse taking.

There are 29 pulses in acupuncture and your practitioner will check all 29 pulses! After that, he or she will also examine your tongue and eyes. The questions they will ask may seem personally invasive and are very intimate, however, it is an integral part of acupuncture. Without a thorough examination and honest answers to the questions, a practitioner is not going to be able to diagnose you correctly or implement your treatment with optimal effects.

THE THEORY OF MERIDIANS IN ACUPUNCTURE

Acupuncture is based on qi ("che") which according to TCM, is an invisible energy that flows throughout the body. This is where the expression yin and yang come from. Put simply, when there is an imbalance in your body, the qi is blocked and you experience a health problem or a disease.

Attempts to relate the meridians' energy patterns in the body have not been conclusive, but interestingly, there is evidence that acupoints have a lower electrical resistance than non-acupuncture sites. Ah, the mystery continues!

EVIDENCE AND RESEARCH

Surprisingly, despite all the unknowns, there have been many studies exploring meridians within the body. In a Spanish study in 1992, radioactive tracers were injected to prove the theory of the meridians. It was discovered that our bodies seem to have a transmission system linked to neurochemicals. This would explain the theory of the meridians. Clearly there is more to our bodies than the circulatory and lymphatic systems. Perhaps, it is our neurochemicals that are affected by acupuncture. Yet, there is a lot we don't know about the body (as much as we hate to admit it).

If you don't like the idea of having needles inserted, there is an alternative, that is, acupressure, which seems to work, but can take longer to achieve results.

During acupressure, cupping is used. In this case, glass cups are placed over acupoints to draw qi and blood towards them. When a practitioner uses cupping, he or she also looks at the colour of the skin. In a healthy person, skin colour returns to normal quickly. However, it can leave some marks as you may have seen on some famous Olympic athletes in recent years.

MEDICAL OPINION ON ACUPUNCTURE

A growing number of doctors now practice acupuncture. It may work by releasing pain-killing and anti-inflammatory endorphins into the blood. It is also a possibility that neurochemicals may go past what is often called "gate control" and deliver messages to the brain that helps to start a recovery or healing process in certain parts of the body. Again, we can't know for sure. But we can theorize!

HOW ACUPUNCTURE CAN BENEFIT YOU IN MENOPAUSE

It is believed that acupuncture can help to balance the endocrine system which controls our hormones. This helps reduce and better control hot flashes, irritability, and insomnia. In fact, 80% of women who tried acupuncture during menopause say they experienced an improvement in symptoms. This is a rather astonishing number and is definitely something to consider when looking into what treatments you might want to try. While none of us are made the same, there is also the law of averages indicating that most future events do assume the average (Don't worry; you've still got your uniqueness. All I'm saying is that acupuncture might be worth a shot for a lot of women.).

There are several acupressure points indicated when using acupuncture. The points used depends on the patient, but the most common points are the kidney, heart, and spleen.

CHAPTER ELEVEN

AROMATHERAPY

Aromatherapy is the use of aromatic plant extracts and essentials oils for healing. It has been around for thousands of years, and modern aromatherapy is largely based on research done in France and Egypt.

In France, essential oils are sometimes prescribed as an alternative to conventional medication. Outside of France, aromatherapy is more popular as an extension of beauty treatments, but there is every possibility that some of the plants used in aromatherapy can transfer their active compounds via their oils. After all, the skin is an organ capable of absorbing what we put on it. From there, compounds may easily enter the bloodstream and have various effects.

THEORY OF AROMATHERAPY

According to modern theory, essential oils are absorbed by the body through the pores when you receive a massage. Alternatively, you can also inhale them. It is believed that the oils can help a person relax and heal. You may have experienced this when exposed to certain scents, like lavender or peppermint. In fact, lavender is a common aroma used for Epsom salt baths due to its relaxation effects.

EVIDENCE AND RESEARCH

According to trials in London in 1994, patients became calmer when massaged using essential oils, specifically lavender and neroli. However, when an ordinary carrier oil was used, the effects were not the same.

This would suggest that aromatherapy does have both physical and psychological effects. More research is needed, but aromatherapy *has* stood the test of time. After all, it was used and recommended in Ancient Egypt. There's got to be something to it if we're still using it thousands of years later!

MEDICAL OPINION ON AROMATHERAPY

As very little medical evidence exists, most doctors are still skeptical when it comes to the health benefits of aromatherapy. On the other hand, they know deep relaxation and regular massages can help you feel calmer and better. What we need to acknowledge is that while there isn't loads of hard scientific evidence, there is every possibility that aromatherapy oils have therapeutic properties and can be beneficial for overall health and well-being.

HOW AROMATHERAPY CAN BENEFIT YOU IN MENOPAUSE

Aromatherapy often involves essential oils extracted from herbs. We certainly know compounds found in essential oils can help us to relax. What scientists are less sure about is if they can affect the endocrine system. In menopause, it is perhaps best to see aromatherapy as a therapy that helps you to relax. The positive effects of relaxation on the endocrine system are well documented.

The endocrine system's response to stress can be extreme in many cases. In fact, it can lead to increased or longer menopausal symptoms. According to Harvard Medical School, stress has a severe effect on the hormone, cortisol. In turn, this can also impact other hormones and various functions within the body.

When you focus on reducing your stress level, you indirectly support your endocrine system. As mentioned earlier, the hormone, cortisol, does not only control stress levels, but it also increases the risk of excess weight gain, primarily caused by blood sugar dysregulation.

The best essential oils for relaxation include lavender and clary sage. Lotus and ylang-ylang are also helpful.

Clary sage is a plant found growing in the Mediterranean area. In Traditional Folk Medicine, it has been used for stress relief, improved digestion, and anti-inflammatory effects. Furthermore, it is believed that it may help to remedy depression.

Today, lavender grows around the world. It is one of the best-documented essential oils and perhaps one of the most popular ones. A couple of drops on your pillow can even help you sleep better. It may also help when it comes to reducing cortisol levels. A study, published in 2010 in the Journal of Ethnopharmacology, suggested that lavender showed stress-reducing effects in rats. While more human studies are needed, this evidence is promising.

Lotus is not one of the most used essential oils. The use of Lotus is more common in the Near and Far East. According to a recent study in India, lotus shows promise when it comes to nerve generation. Therefore, there is every possibility that it may affect stress levels positively. Lotus is also known to have some health benefits when inhaled. We know rosemary can affect us when inhaled, but we are still waiting for scientific evidence that indicates lotus works in a similar way.

A 2006 study indicated that another herb ylang-ylang has a relaxing effect when it is absorbed through the skin. This is a user-friendly herb with few recorded side effects.

CHAPTER TWELVE

HOMEOPATHY & NATUROPATHY

"Homeopathy cures a larger percentage of cases than any other method of treatment and is beyond doubt safer and more economical."

- Mahatma Gandhi (1869-1948)

Homeopathy was developed in the 18th century and is based on the idea of "like cures like." The logic behind homeopathy sounds a bit odd, but there is a basis for this concept. A substance that may cause illness in a healthy person may cure a person who is not healthy. These substances are diluted many times to make a remedy that is safe (And when you think about it, not to bring up a controversial topic, but this kind of works similarly to many vaccines).

Homeopathy is well-established in Europe and India. In addition, it is growing in popularity in the United States. Thus, it may be worth exploring for combatting menopausal symptoms.

THEORY OF HOMEOPATHY

The body is said to be controlled by a vital force that maintains its state of health. In homeopathy, illness or a health condition is seen as the body's attempt at self-healing.

Homeopathy seeks to promote self-healing instead of dealing with symptoms (aka it gets to the root of the problem or tries to anyway!). The name says it all. Home is derived from the Greek word "homolos" meaning "same." The second part of homeopathy comes from the word "pathos" which means "suffering." Throw them together and you get "same suffering" which reads very similar to "like cures like."

EVIDENCE AND RESEARCH

There is some evidence that homeopathy works. The British Medical Journal published a study in 1994 which indicated that homeopathy treatments were successful. Patients took part in a double-blind trial of homeopathy for asthma and allergies and the results were impressive. As patients did not know if they were receiving a remedy or a placebo, personal opinions could not influence the outcome. Yet, again, it's always a statistics game. More research is needed to solidify these claims.

MEDICAL OPINION

Current medical therapy can't explain how homeopathy works. However, a growing number of doctors around the world are training in homeopathy.

It seems homeopathy can often offer a cure where conventional medicine has failed. This has been experienced by *both* patients and doctors alike.

HOW HOMEOPATHY CAN BENEFIT YOU IN MENOPAUSE

There are thousands of homeopathy remedies. When it comes to menopause, two of the most frequently indicated and used remedies are rock salt and Sepia.

Sepia is well-documented to help remedy depression and excess perspiration. It is these two benefits that homeopaths suggest Sepia as a remedy in menopause. If you are experiencing hot flashes and feeling blue, Sepia may be worth trying for 3 days.

Rock salt also shows promise as a remedy for menopause. If you are experiencing fatigue, it can help to balance your body again and maybe even give you more energy. There is an increasing number of indications that Himalayan rock salt can help to relieve menopausal symptoms due to its' potential natural ability to help our bodies realize an increased need to replenish certain minerals.

THE THEORY OF NATUROPATHY

Naturopathy is also known as natural medicine. It was developed in the 19th century and is founded on the principle that the body can heal itself. Naturopaths follow the principle that the body's natural state is in equilibrium. This state can be disturbed by an unhealthy lifestyle or other influencing factors such as pollution.

Naturopaths look for underlying causes rather than treating symptoms. They combine diet, supplements, and non-invasive therapies to stimulate healing. By now, you might notice a bit of a theme with these alternative therapies; they all strive to work with your body rather than adding more fuel to the fire.

Overall, naturopaths take a multi-faceted approach to healing and natural resources. Wholefoods, fresh air, and water are all important aspects of this form of complementary medicine. The idea is to achieve homeostasis, which means all things are equal. Once again, one of the main principles behind naturopathy is a vital life force.

EVIDENCE AND RESEARCH

We know that foods contain a wide variety of antioxidants, vitamins, and minerals that we need to stay healthy, hence, it is only reasonable to say that what we eat has an impact on our health. For instance, scientists have found a range of antioxidants in food that can help us to combat disease. Additionally, vitamin or mineral deficiencies can have serious impacts on our health and wellness.

MEDICAL OPINION

Many long-held beliefs of naturopathy are practiced by doctors. A fiber-rich diet and fresh food is recommended, similar to what many conventional doctors recommend. Stress management and exercise are key factors here as well that can help you to lead a better and healthier life. While these topics might be discussed quite frequently in the health industry, they are actually the very foundations of naturopathy (and for a good reason!). At the end of the day, much disease and suffering in the Western world (not all) may come down to a lack of doing the basics, like regular exercise and relaxation.

NUTRITIONAL THERAPIES AS PART OF NATUROPATHY

Are we what we eat? In the next part of this book, we will talk about food and nutrition. However, both conventional and alternative medicine believe that what we eat has a strong link to our general health. A range of nutritional therapies was developed in the early part of the 20th century. They embrace a wide range of approaches to both special diets and supplements. So, let's take a closer look.

HOW CAN NATUROPATHY BENEFIT YOU DURING MENOPAUSE

During menopause, naturopathy can be used to guide you in the right direction. The idea behind naturopathy is a range of herbal remedies. It is also important to realize (if you haven't already) that dietary recommendations play an important part in naturopathy.

Managing menopause naturally, using a range of practices associated with naturopathy may have many advantages for women who are sensitive to conventional HRT. According to the popular site, NCBI, naturopathy has a place during menopause. It can help to reduce symptoms including hot flashes, irritability, and insomnia. To get the most out of naturopathy, you should visit a qualified practitioner who can tailor a plan to your specific needs and goals.

CHAPTER THIRTEEN

WESTERN HERBALISM

"Let food be thy medicine and medicine be thy food."

- Hippocrates

Did you know that it is estimated that over 85% of the world relies on herbs for health? We take them as part of a supplement routine and use them when we cook food. Many conventional drugs and medicines are based on herbs. In the past 300 years, plant species from Europe, North America, Africa, and many other parts of the world have become part of Western Herbalism.

THE THEORY OF SYNERGY

When we talk about herbalism, the concept of synergy is often mentioned. Herbalists believe that a mix of leaves, flowers, stalks, and roots creates synergy. It means the therapeutic effect is greater when they are used together rather than separately. In short, this concept represents the major difference between herbalism and conventional medicine.

EVIDENCE AND RESEARCH

The evidence to support the claims made by herbalists is growing fast. The positive effects of many herbs can be as strong as conventional medicine. In Europe, claims made by herbal products need to be backed up by scientific research. It is thought that a Natural Medicine Directive may be introduced in the United States and other countries before too long. This may help cut through confusion regarding this medicine, as well as potentially help people take it a tad more seriously.

Herbs that have been proven to have scientific benefits are Echinacea, garlic, ginger, Gingko, saw palmetto, and St John's Wort.

MEDICAL OPINION

Although, many doctors still view herbs as outdated health solutions, they are beginning to realize the need for more research. After all, the flower, digitalis, is used to treat heart disease. Furthermore, many synthetic preparations have been made from herbs by coping active compounds found in herbs. However, it is also important to appreciate that herbs can have side effects, and they are definitely something to look into before consuming any kind of herb.

If you are experiencing menopausal symptoms for which you can't find relief using a conventional medication, herbs may be worth considering. When you are new to using herbs, it is best not to self-medicate. Instead, visit a qualified herbalist or doctor who is happy to prescribe herbal remedies.

THE BEST HERBAL SUPPLEMENTS FOR MENOPAUSE

Some of the best herbal remedies for menopause may include:

* Red Clover

* Black Cohosh

* Dong Quai

* Evening Primrose oil

* Ginseng

RED CLOVER

Red clover is a legume plant. This may mean it has similarities with soy. From what we know, soy does contain isoflavones and plant-based estrogens. It is the way we process soy and add it to our food that may cause negative health problems including cancer.

As with many herbal remedies, studies are needed to understand it better. However, according to popular opinion, many women have experienced positive results when using red clover. It may help you to better manage hot flashes, fatigue, and sleep disturbances experienced during menopause.

BLACK COHOSH

Black Cohosh is a popular plant-based supplement when it comes to combating menopausal symptoms. A range of health benefits have been noted. Many women who use this popular supplement have not only reported a reduction in hot flashes and problems with insomnia but have also reported that other health problems associated with menopause such as vaginal dryness, depression, and irritability seem to be reduced after taking Black Cohosh for some time.

Compared to many other supplements associated with menopause, it is one of the safer supplements. To date, no serious negative side effects and contra-indications have been recorded.

DONG QUAI

Dong Quai is a Chinese herb that has long been used in TCM and Chinese herbalism. Not only can it help to reduce the symptoms of menopause, but Western researchers are also beginning to think it may have compounds that can help with chronic inflammation.

According to Mount Sinai, Dong Quai has been used for at least one thousand years as a tonic in both China and Japan. Today, it is still one of the most popular herbs used in TCM.

Practitioners of Chinese Herbalism use the herb to remedy problems with women's reproductive health and heavy periods. It's kind of a no-brainer, then, why some women may experience benefits with its use during menopause.

Occasionally, you may hear Don Quai called the "female ginseng." There are relatively few studies, but it seems that the herb can have positive effects from premenstrual problems to menopausal ones. This indicates that it influences the endocrine system. Hence, it may be worth trying if you are experiencing hot flashes or other severe symptoms. As per usual (are we noticing a theme here?), more studies are needed.

EVENING PRIMROSE OIL

Evening primrose oil is derived from the flower of the same name. Although there are indications that they may help to combat breast pain, there is scarce information and evidence when it comes to its positive health effects. Many claim that evening primrose oil helps to balance the hormones, but there is no evidence for that. However, this could be true. If you are using conventional HRT, it is not recommended to use this herb as it is believed to possibly disrupt HRT.

One thing we do know is that it contains an anti-inflammatory compound called gamma-linoleic acid, which is known to remedy skin conditions. This flower seems to be particularly useful when it comes to psoriasis. Evening primrose oil is typically available as a topical remedy.

GINSENG

Scientists think that ginseng may have the ability to stimulate or synthesize estrogen activity in the body. This means that when you use this popular Chinese herb, you are less likely to experience hot flashes and other symptoms. A published Chinese study involving experiments with mice given ginseng showed that their estrogen levels may have increased after their ovaries were removed. However, no conclusive evidence has been found. Still, many women claim that they have experienced positive side effects when they use ginseng as a supplement.

When you read about herbs for menopause, you often see soy and flax seeds listed. Technically, they are not herbs but are medicinal plants instead. Soy is often claimed to be a life changer and attributed to a lower incidence of menopausal symptoms in Asian women. This may not be true, however, there is a chance that seaweed helps as it offers a better explanation; Iodine and other compounds found in seaweed support a healthy thyroid. This link between seaweed and the thyroid, which influences menopause, is justified.

HOW WESTERN HERBALISM CAN BENEFIT YOU IN MENOPAUSE

Western Herbalism is also occasionally called Traditional Folk Medicine. Both wise women and monks were early practitioners of Western Herbalism. In the early days of Western Herbalism, menopause wasn't recognized. It stands to reason that many early herbal practitioners did not know about hormones. At the same time, it must be said that women's troubles were often referenced, and it would seem practitioners recognized the change.

The best traditional herbal remedy that has been mentioned is perhaps red clover. As science has progressed, there are indications that red clover contains natural isoflavones, which are plant-based chemicals that can produce estrogen-like effects in the body. It is thought that isoflavones have a positive effect on osteoporosis and hot flashes. It's also thought that these compounds have anti-inflammatory effects, giving way to various health benefits.

CHAPTER FOURTEEN

SUPPLEMENTS AND VITAMINS

"The body is a temple, but it's also a laboratory, and vitamins are the tools we use to keep it running properly."

- Terri Guillemets

Every day, one in three adults take a supplement; many do so in hopes that they are going to make them healthy. Aren't we all looking for that "miracle pill" for anti-aging and good health?

The supplement industry is worth billions upon billions of dollars. All forms of supplements are popular from mineral supplements to herbal supplements. We often choose to only consider vitamins as supplements. However, in theory, vitamins are not supplements – they are just vitamins.

However, it's important to note that the purpose of a "supplement" is within the name. Supplements should *supplement* what you're already doing, not serve as a be-all, end-all solution.

WHO NEEDS A SUPPLEMENT?

Where specific requirements are not met by what we eat, we may need to take a supplement. Women often benefit from taking supplements at various stages in their life. But when it comes to supplements, there are different schools of thought.

More recently, we have come to realize that even though we eat healthy food, what we eat may not give us all the nutritional values we need. The way we produce and transport food are two of the contributing factors to our food lacking what we need to stay healthy. In other words, the food we eat today (even some whole foods) don't contain as much vitamin or mineral content as they once did.

Much of our food is produced using advanced practices. Vegetables, fruits, and berries are often grown hydroponically. This means they only get the nutrients they are "fed." The result is often a loss of many of the valuable vitamins and minerals we need to stay healthy.

Meat and fish are often farmed. As they don't live their lives in a natural environment, they don't have access to essential vitamins and minerals they may need to produce healthy food. We also add things to animal meat production, which includes everything from animal feed supplements to hormones for the animal to grow faster. What you need to remember is that all of this is passed down the food chain to us.

As food is transported over long distances, its nutritional value is lost in transit. Pollution also affects the plants that produce our food. This leads to lower nutritional values.

Thus, the need for supplementation may be on the rise. However, we should always work to get the basics down first, then use supplements to compliment our foundational habits and dietary choices or availability.

PROCEED WITH CAUTION

Does this mean you should take a supplement? The supplement industry likes to sell you all sorts of supplements, so if you are thinking about taking a supplement, it is best to check your vitamin and mineral levels. After all, the supplement industry aims to make money. Myths and misconceptions are *common*. If you have symptoms indicating a deficiency, why not speak to your doctor first? You can easily spend a lot of money on supplements that you don't need.

Bear in mind that you can overdose on supplements and vitamins if it is not controlled. For instance, vitamins D and A are fat-soluble vitamins. They are stored by the body and build up if you take too much. Fortunately, a doctor can easily check if you are low in vitamin D or A.

The members of the vitamin B group are water-soluble. It means they are not stored by the body. We need to take in a certain amount of vitamin B every day to stay healthy. As far as supplements go, this is one of the best supplements you can take. Vitamin B plays a vital role in almost all functions in the body. Taking one single B vitamin, for instance, B12, does not benefit you. The members of this vitamin group work together. Therefore, for menopausal treatments and remedies, having a good level of vitamin B is very important.

THE BEST VITAMINS FOR MENOPAUSE

A vitamin B supplement is one of the best supplements you can take when you are experiencing menopausal symptoms. The most crucial B vitamins are B6 and B12.

Vitamin B6 helps with energy production in the body and supports healthy blood cells, while Vitamin B12 helps to form healthy cells including blood cells. Vitamin C on the other hand is a vital antioxidant. One of the best natural sources of vitamin C is apples and grapefruit. Although oranges contain vitamin C, they also contain a high amount of citric acid which is associated with aches and pains in the joints during menopause. As it is such a vital antioxidant, taking a vitamin C supplement is an excellent idea.

At the same time, don't fix what isn't broken. If you're able to get plenty of vitamin C (such as strawberries, bell peppers, and oranges) and vitamin B (eggs, meat, citrus fruit, dairy products, and leafy greens) in your diet as it is, you might have no need for supplementation. In fact, obtaining these nutrients in your diet is a much better option since the body is primed to absorb these nutrients in their natural form with ease.

OTHER SUPPLEMENTS FOR MENOPAUSE

Mineral supplements are also important in menopause. A daily calcium supplement helps to support your bone health. You may also consider taking a potassium supplement. Potassium helps to maintain healthy levels of fluid inside the cells. A low potassium level contributes to bloating and weight gain. But yet again, you can get these from your diet. Dairy isn't usually something to be feared, and it contains plenty of calcium. Potassium, on the other hand, can be obtained via your diet by eating more bananas, oranges, and potatoes. Remember, a whole foods diet goes a long way!

Apart from mineral supplements, you may also want to consider an Omega 3 fatty acid supplement. However, if you are taking blood thinning drugs including aspirin, you should limit your intake of Omega 3 to 500mg per day. Furthermore, omega 3 can be obtained from various seafood and plant oils.

TAKING SUPPLEMENTS

Many say that they don't get any benefit from supplements. This may be true because the way you take your supplements matters. Since the body considers supplements as food, it means the body needs time to digest them and may need other vitamins or minerals to adequately absorb and use them.

So, if you do decide to opt for supplements due to availability of food or a deficiency, how should you take them? This may depend on the supplement. Some digest and absorb better alongside food, and others don't. It may also be beneficial to take supplements 20 minutes before breakfast since the body is primed for nutrient absorption. But, again, this may depend. Ensure you discuss with your pharmacist or doctor the best way to take the supplement you've been recommended.

CHAPTER FIFTEEN

MOVEMENT THROUGH MENOPAUSE

"When I asked for a smoking hot body, menopause was not what I had in mind."

- Unknown

Maintaining a healthy weight is important at any age, and especially during menopause. When you carry excess weight, your body naturally produces more estrogen. Inevitably, this can lead to increased or worse menopausal symptoms. On top of this, hormonal variances during menopause can make weight loss tricky, as well as lead to weight gain. Yet, this doesn't mean that maintaining a healthy weight is impossible. In fact, most of this all comes down to doing the basics such as eating a healthy diet, getting enough sleep, and exercising regularly.

Ultimately, many factors play a role when it comes to weight management. While not all women gain weight during menopause, many women do. In fact, increasing belly fat is one of the main complaints of women approaching or going through menopause. Luckily, there's a few things you can do about it but first, before we dive into the exercise side of things, let's examine more closely why this happens in the first place.

REASONS FOR WEIGHT GAIN IN MENOPAUSE

Hormonal imbalances are the primary reasons for gaining weight during the menopausal years (Ah, hormones again!). The most common hormones at play here are estrogen, testosterone, progesterone, and cortisol (possibly no surprise there). A reduction of the main three hormones–estrogen, testosterone, and progesterone–leads to an increase in the production of cortisol, also known as the stress hormone.

It wasn't until recently that researchers started to dive further into the effects of cortisol on the body. Put simply, cortisol increases when we experience physical or mental stress. On the mental side of things, this is often referred to as the "fight-or-flight" response. However, in many cases of mental stress, this response doesn't disappear once the threat has gone. In the modern world, we have various stressors and societal pressures causing cortisol to run rampant in the body. When one hormone increases, it impacts all the others and creates hormonal imbalances.

When the level of cortisol is increased, we start piling on weight. The most common areas where weight gain occurs is around the midsection, tummy, hips, and upper thighs. Bra fat, or back fat, and extra fat around the armpit areas are not unusual either.

Now, this happens for a few reasons. The production of cortisol depletes vitamin C. Chronic stress also depletes various other nutrients, such as magnesium, zinc, and more. So, what happens when we need to replenish these nutrients? We experience *cravings*. But sometimes we read the signals wrong. We chose unhealthy, easy, and convenient options. Most often, these options are high in calories and low in multiple nutrients, meaning we end up eating more.

On top of this, unfortunately, many of us fall flat on our face when trying to lose a little bit of weight via fad or quick-fix diets. Maybe we do lose weight or we don't. But most of the time, we end up gaining more weight as we get caught up in an epic restrict-binge cycle. So many women have gone through the throes of restrictive dieting. The most common pitfall? After days of restriction, we binge eat. We shame ourselves. And then we do the whole cycle over again. However, there is a way to do this better and break free from the "diet" craze. Of course, if you have disordered eating, you should seek out professional help when needed. Yet, a lot of this comes down to balance with diet and exercise.

You don't have to be perfect but the 80-20 rule says it all. Aim for 80% perfection and 20% of slack. And don't overburden your body either. Too much exercise or too much junk food will interfere with good health and weight loss. However, just the right amount of exercise and a treat now and again will keep you on track with your health, menopausal symptoms, and overall life satisfaction. More on this coming up!

At the end of the day, a combination of the right diet and exercise is important to combat fatty deposits. Increasingly, researchers are beginning to appreciate that aerobic exercise alone does not combat excess fat and weight gain in menopause. So, what does? Let's dig deeper!

DIFFERENT TYPES OF BELLY FAT

First, let's take a slight detour. During menopause you can put on different types of fat in and around your stomach. Subcutaneous fat is the kind of fat that you find directly underneath the skin. Subcutaneous fatty deposits are soft. You can reduce them by doing exercise and eating a balanced diet.

The other type of belly fat, which many women experience in menopause, is visceral fat. This fat is found deeper inside the belly and surrounds the organ. Doctors often call this "the dangerous belly fat." It is associated with a range of health conditions including digestive disorders and diseases affecting the uterus and the ovaries.

To the touch, visceral fat feels hard and may even lead to your belly button sticking out. Getting rid of visceral fat is more challenging. You need to pay close attention to your daily activity level and diet to get rid of it. In fact, visceral fat may indicate you need to make more drastic changes to your lifestyle, including altering your diet, getting sufficient sleep, reducing stress, and sticking to a regular exercise routine. But with any new habit, it's a little bit at a time. Small steps lead to big changes. Plus, paying attention to these aspects of your lifestyle also contribute to better and more balanced hormones. It's a win-win really!

EXERCISING DURING MENOPAUSE

Not only does exercise help you with weight management, but it also has a range of other health benefits. Regular exercise and daily movement can further help prevent osteoporosis and help you gain more energy. So, let's break this done a bit further.

WHAT KIND OF EXERCISE SHOULD YOU DO?

While some exercises are therapeutic, high-impact exercises may do more harm than good. When you are experiencing joint pain, you should stay away from certain exercises. On top of this, if you're overly stressed, doing long bouts of HIIT is a sure-fire way to take your stress levels to another level. Not good. Yet, at the same time, small bouts of HIIT can have its place when improving overall health and longevity during and after menopause.

Overall, most types of exercise help to build both healthy bones and muscles. Many types further can help lower your stress levels (but again, the wrong type at the wrong time can increase them too!). Along with dieting, exercising is one of the most important things you can do in menopause for better health. Doctors agree that exercise and a healthy diet are key factors when it comes to controlling and reducing menopause symptoms, including maintaining a healthy weight. In the following sections, we take closer look at the types of exercise you should consider during menopause. And one quick note here: if you're new to exercise, aim to find something you enjoy. The type of exercise here matters less since doing *something* is always better than doing nothing.

AEROBIC ACTIVITY

Aerobic activity, also referred to as cardio, helps to boost circulation and enhances heart health. Aerobics first became popular when Jane Fonda encouraged us to get more physical in the 1980s (along with various pop tunes with a similar name). Since then, aerobics have evolved into a variety of different aerobic options to choose from. When it comes to aerobics, you truly are spoiled for choice. You can choose step aerobics, low-impact aerobics, or just a mixed aerobics class. In fact, low-impact aerobics offers many of the same benefits as more intense aerobic workouts such as step and high impact.

However, don't feel as though you need to sign up for a bunch of aerobic classes. If keeping it simple works, keep it simple! Go for a few quick walks around the block. Or take a hike on the weekend with friends. Do what works for you. No one expects you to go for a 10-mile run each day. In fact, you shouldn't. This will probably just add layers of stress, potentially exacerbating menopausal symptoms. Again, keep it simple. Think about doing this type of activity to improve your heart and respiratory health or as a way to socialize with friends. You can even take work calls out on a walk if it suits your schedule! Heck, even walking your dog enough each day might meet your "aerobics" quota and reap the same benefits.

Alternatively, for those with painful joints, swimming is another wonderful aerobic exercise. You can also choose between a variety of swimming styles. Breaststroke is popular and offers many benefits when it comes to toning the body. Doing the crawl, backstroke, and butterfly lets you work on different muscle groups Swimming is often overlooked but it has heaps of benefits similar to other cardio options without the joint strain.

WALKING

Walking is a great exercise you can do anywhere with next to no equipment. And yes, walking deserves its very own section!

Did you know that some of the fittest people are dog walkers? A dog walker may walk several times per day. If you walk fast, you can burn about 10 calories per minute. Most walkers burn about 5 calories per minute. It is great for cardiac function. Many studies on walking are ongoing. When we look at our bodies, we can see that they have joints. Scientists believe that this means we were meant to walk. The human body has not changed very much since we walked our way from the plains of Africa. In fact, we haven't evolved much past our hunter-gatherer ancestors, which indicates the body is made to move! The science even suggests we *thrive* with movement, in particular little bits of walking throughout our day. And going even further, we tend to age faster and succumb to various diseases when we assume a mostly sedentary lifestyle.

If you look around your local area, you will probably find that there are many walking clubs. Join in and you will benefit from exercise and social activities. You could also walk to catch up with friends. You don't even need to do one big walk. It could be little walks sprinkled throughout your day (In fact, this might be better for you!). All in all, walking enhances bone strength, improves muscle mass, improves heart and respiratory health, and so much more. In menopause, walking has even been shown to combat the symptoms of fatigue and brain fog.

On top of this, walking in the morning or evening can kill two birds with one stone. How so? Well, for those with sleep troubles, you'll want to listen up! Walking in the morning or evening exposes the neurons in our eyes to certain light rays from the sun. This can help regulate our circadian rhythm via the suppression and stimulation of specific hormones involved in these processes. In turn, it might just help you get a better night's rest (Light and movement count for a lot here!).

Overall, there is some truth to that 10 000 steps per day phenomenon. Most experts agree this is a good goal to have. Yet, if you don't already walk each day, start small and slowly build. Going too hard, too soon is never encouraged!

HIIT TRAINING

HIIT stands for High Intensity Interval Training, which is a way of both intensifying and alternating training methods. You switch between periods of high intensity to periods of rest. When you are exercising at high intensity, you will often feel exhausted before your brief period of rest. Weights and bands are often used to make the high-intensity part of the workout more challenging.

HIIT is a great way of elevating the heart rate and burning more calories. On top of that, HIIT workouts challenge the body. HIIT is also a great way to build resilience, mentally and physically. However, by no means should you do a 60 minute HIIT session each day. Gone are the days when this is the general recommendation. Instead, aim for one to two, 10–20-minute HIIT sessions every 7-10 days. This will help you gain the benefits but also won't overburden the body.

Additionally, don't perform HIIT if you feel overly stress, fatigued, or exhausted. Again, this will increase cortisol causing more issues. Listening to your body is always key with exercise!

Alternatively, if you are tight on time, interval workouts, similar to HIIT, offer some solutions. You don't necessarily have to switch between high and low intensity. Rather, you can use similar intervals to perform different sets of exercise. For example, you could do squats and lunges and other leg movements for a quick 15–20-minute workout. Remember, something is always better than nothing. But if your body needs rest, let it rest! Rest days are just as important as your workout days. It's all about balance!

PILATES

Pilates was founded a hundred years ago by Joseph Pilates to help ballerinas and dancers strengthen their bodies. Traditionally, it is done on a reformer bed which has a bed and springs, ropes, and pulleys for resistance. Reformer Pilates focuses on your using your core to strengthen your belly, hips, shoulders, and arms. It is a great overall low impact exercise.

Pilates is gentle, but at the same time, it offers an excellent workout. To benefit from Pilates, you need to be consistent with your classes. Attending classes, a couple of times per week helps you to keep up with the technique and the movements.

Pilates provides a gentler way to move during menopause. Once, it was considered an exercise only for dancers, but now, Pilates has become more mainstream. It has been recognized that Pilates help to soothe tension in the neck and shoulders. Women who experience cramps in their legs and arms during menopause say that Pilates has helped them as well. It can help to prevent muscle, tendon, and ligament injuries.

It is also well-recognized that Pilates helps to improve posture. That is why it is so popular with dancers. Pilates is about technique, so be patient with yourself and you will benefit. Try it out! This could be a great option for you, especially if you're someone who is prone to injuries or has past injuries.

WEIGHTLIFTING

Here's the big one, weightlifting is the exercise that almost every guru, expert, and doctor alike agrees on as being highly beneficial as we age and especially advantageous during menopause. According to Harvard Medical School, strength training helps to improve bone density. In fact, it may even improve bone density more than aerobic exercises such as jogging and riding a bicycle. It also leads to better flexibility. If we lose our flexibility, we risk becoming frail and increase our chances of falls.

Many women may worry about weightlifting as they think they are going to end up with large muscles or look "bulky." This is yet another persistent myth that has very little foundation to it.

For example, one pound of muscle takes up much less space than one pound of fat. When you gain muscle, you actually "tone" and "slim" down the body. Plus, to get "bulky," you'd have to be putting in some serious hours in the gym. It takes a lot of work to get there, and gaining healthy muscle usually doesn't make one bigger or "bulky." The most toned women you see actually have the most muscle!

Weightlifting has many benefits apart from improving your muscle strength; it can help to improve your bone strength and cardiac function. Added to that, it benefits your posture and balance. To make sure you get the maximum benefits from weightlifting, you should do it at least three times per week. This ensures you are maintaining or gaining muscle as opposed to losing it.

On top of this, you want to progressively overload when you lift. This means that your lifts should be hard! If you're able to do 20 reps easily enough, you're not lifting heavy enough. The last one to two reps of any movement should be tough. We want to be almost pushing our muscles to failure. This will cause adequate muscle breakdown, which means on those rest days, your body will be working hard to adequately build up new muscle! Inevitably, diet is a big part of all of this. We need enough protein to drive muscle growth. We'll talk more about diet later on.

If you're unsure where to start with weightlifting, it's highly encouraged to invest in a coach or personal trainer. Getting the proper form and technique down pat is essential to reap the benefits and avoid injury.

RECOVERY MOVEMENT AND TOOLS

Rest is important and should never be underestimated. However, rest doesn't mean dropping everything and curling up on the couch for days on end. Long durations of sedentary behavior are never good. In fact, your "rest days," such as breaks from planned and more intense workouts, should include some form of gentle movement. Walking daily is highly encouraged for various health benefits, but you can also do the following types of other exercises and activities. Many of the following can also help reduce stress and tension throughout the body, helping you to truly relax.

YOGA

You should not underestimate the health benefits of yoga. It works on the mind as well as the body. When you practice yoga, you become more aware of how you feel in your mind, and you enhance the mind-body connection. That being said, you don't have to be into meditation to benefit from yoga. You can enjoy yoga just as much when you think of it as a way of exercising.

If you go to a yoga class, you will soon discover social benefits. Yogis are often friendly and like to socialize after class. If you are not sociable, you can practice yoga at home. There are several good YouTube Channels and Facebook streaming services. But, if you have never done yoga before, it is a good idea to try at least a couple of classes.

There is little wonder why yoga has become popular. First, you have a range of different yoga styles to choose from. Also, don't forget about spin-offs and other complementary ways of exercising that can be added to yoga, including meditation and visualization.

Yoga is a popular way to increase flexibility and core strength without doing high impact exercises. As a form of exercise, it increases flexibility and gently builds muscles. If you are experiencing stiffness and back pain, yoga is one of the exercises you should try. It also benefits you in other ways apart from the physical ones. Most women who practice yoga say that it helps them with anxiety and depression. If you are not sleeping well, you should consider going to yoga regularly. Breathing exercises (pranas) are an integral part of yoga, and can help damper the stress response, giving you a much needed break from the chaos of your day-to-day.

Lastly, yin yoga is a form of restorative yoga that can be significant on rest days between weightlifting sessions. This type of yoga stretches the body and gives you space to relax and de-stress. Look up yoga classes in your area. Give them a try and see how you feel afterward.

MEDITATION

Meditation is a mental discipline that is an essential part of many world religions. Many priests even regard prayer as a form of meditation. The intention of meditation is to induce profound relaxation and increased awareness at the same time. A variety of techniques can be used to achieve a meditative state. What we know about meditation is that it reduces the body's fight-or-flight response.

During meditation, a state of deep relaxation is experienced. We know that this happens as we have been able to measure brain activity in the cortex part of the brain. This activity can be analyzed and chartered. Significant psychological and physical benefits are linked to the brainwave patterns that take place during meditation.

We know that meditation produces a different set of alpha waves in the brain. This has been proven by measuring brain waves under clinical conditions. In fact, an increasing number of doctors think that meditation may be just as important as physical exercise and diet. It has been shown that meditation helps to control blood pressure and our breath patterns. As a result, many doctors recommend meditation as a therapy or regular mental practice.

It's really easy to start meditation nowadays as well. There an abundant of resources, including meditation options of YouTube and even phone apps, like Headspace or Insight Timer, that have various types of meditations to choose from.

VISUALIZATION

The technique is said to help one cope with stress. It can also be a powerful tool for achieving your goals. Visualization first came to light in the 1970s when psychologists discovered that visualizing treatment goals helped many patients. Patients that are overcome by physical and mental problems often find it hard to understand the outcome of a specific situation. The therapy can be very relaxing and creative at the same time. Interestingly, similar studies have been conducted on professional athletes where visualization as proven to be a powerful tool in achieving the outcome they want in their sport of choice.

Today, we often talk about manifestation. In many ways, this is just a re-branding of recognized visualization techniques.

While it remains unclear how visualization works, it *is* clear that it increases activity in the right hemisphere of the brain. This is the part of the brain relating to feelings and emotions. Research using emission photography scans has shown that imagery involving sight activates the brain. Most specifically, it activates the cerebral cortex. In some way, this is how visualization can produce such powerful effects! Visualization is sometimes part of meditation and is practiced in yoga.

A vivid image can be sent from the brain using the hormonal system. It both helps to control and calm down the heart rate and other body functions. Try visualizing where you want to be a few months from now. Make sure to include plenty of details here by engaging all of your senses. This can help path the way toward this becoming your reality, such as having fewer or even non menopausal symptoms! Obviously, action will also count for a lot. Yet, visualization shouldn't go underestimated.

CHAPTER SIXTEEN

DIETARY CONSIDERATIONS FOR MENOPAUSE

"People who love to eat are always the best people."
- Julia Child

In menopause, the digestion system may seem to have a mind of its own. Perhaps no matter what you eat, an upset stomach or indigestion tends to follow, no doubt posing various challenges. Yet, the digestion of food and elimination of waste products are the cornerstones of health (and hormonal harmony!). In fact, many autoimmune conditions are linked to problems within the digestive tract.

When the body is deprived of certain nutrients, it becomes ill. If it can't eliminate toxins (which includes "used" or broken down hormones), illness may also develop. A balanced diet and low stress levels are important for both our digestive and excretory functions. Potentially unsurprisingly, everything in the body is connected!

A well-balanced mind and body are often a result of a healthy lifestyle. Diet is very much a part of that. We call some foods, superfoods. The truth is that even the humble apple is a superfood. And digging even deeper, whole foods, like fruits and veggies, all deserve this badge of honor. When we steer clear of processed and pre-packaged food items, our health improves.

Gradually, more doctors are beginning to appreciate that diet plays a crucial role in reducing menopausal symptoms and treating disease. However, *some* doctors are skeptical when it comes to the benefits of diet as far as the treatment of disease goes. At the same time, it is believed that certain diets can help us to reduce the likelihood of disease and maybe even control health conditions.

There are many popular diets today. We have all heard of diets such as Keto, Paleo, and Intermittent Fasting. The question is, are they right for menopause? Well, the truth is that most of these popular diets aren't fit for the perimenopause, menopausal, or postmenopausal woman. In fact, for most, dietary restrictions tend to make things much worse. So, instead, let's take a closer look at what you should turn your attention to when it comes to your diet during menopause (and why!).

EATING WHOLE FOODS FOR BETTER HEALTH

Sure, there's Keto. There's Paleo. There's going Vegan. And all diets have pros and cons. (Nothing against them!) For instance, Keto and Paleo might help someone lose weight. Primarily, this happens due to caloric restriction. Yet, the thing is many of these diets don't help you sustain it. In reality, most women struggle to do Keto or "clean eating" for too long. We end up craving and binging (as mentioned previously in this book).

Thus, a better way to approach your diet is by focusing on inclusion as opposed to exclusion. Fill up on whole foods, like veggies, fruits, nuts, seeds, dairy products, and grass-fed meats. Quality matters here! While this may not be accessible for everyone, you always want to strive for the least processed food possible. This helps lessen chemicals and toxins (no matter how small) from your health. Eating more "real" foods instead of processed and pre-packaged items, will do your body, mind, and menopausal symptoms tons of good. On top of this, your gut health and microbiome will thank you! The gut thrives off these whole foods due to their fiber and polyphenol content, which your gut bacteria loves.

So, what foods should you be focusing on? Let's go a layer deeper, shall we?

PROTEIN

Protein, along with carbs and fats, is a macronutrient. This is where our calories (energy) come from.

Yet, here's a hard truth: most women don't get enough protein. We need at least 90 grams of protein, preferably 0.8 grams of protein per kilogram of bodyweight. And during menopause, this can actually be slightly more, especially if you're strength training since protein drives muscle growth.

This doesn't have to be overly complicated. Common foods like beef, chicken, eggs, nuts, fish, oysters, Greek yogurt, and more, can cover your protein intake. The general rule of thumb here is to try to include 20-30 grams of protein with each meal or snack. This will also help regulate blood sugar levels, which is crucial for lowering stress and inflammation in the body (more on this in a bit).

CALCIUM

Menopausal women, unfortunately, tend to experience significant bone loss. This can lead to osteoporosis (brittle bones and a low bone density), meaning you could be at risk of fractures and breaks.

But this is where calcium plays a valuable role. Getting enough of this mineral is crucial to maintain bone mass and prevent bone loss. On top of this, strength training and regular walks can help prevent bone loss since this signals to the body to generate new bone.

While you can obtain calcium from supplementation, a better way is to get it straight from your diet. If you can tolerate it, milk is one of nature's most perfect foods with a great balance of protein, fats, and carbs. However, there is also cheese, yogurt, and some leafy greens that are also high in calcium. Most women should aim for at least 1200 mg per day of calcium.

OMEGA-3s

Omega-3s are widely known for their contribution to improved brain health, as well as their potential to reduce depression. They also have anti-inflammatory properties, which can help combat menopausal symptom, such as brain fog or mood fluctuations.

A few foods you might want to consider including more of in your diet that are high in omega-3s include salmon, sardines, mackerel, walnuts, flaxseeds, and chia seeds.

B VITAMINS

B vitamins are important for everyone. For the menopausal woman, however, they can help combat fatigue and improve energy production. In turn, this can further help tackle symptoms of depression that may occur during this time.

Foods high in the B vitamins include eggs, chicken, seafood, dairy products, seeds, potatoes, and leafy greens. There are also so many ways to add these to your diet. Get creative. Try new recipes. Have fun with this! When you nourish your body properly, you lay the foundations for good health and a happy and satisfying life. (And likely fewer menopausal symptoms. All wins.)

MAGNESIUM

Here's a little backstory on magnesium: This is actually one mineral none of us get enough of. And it isn't really our fault. More so, this might come down to the lower quality of our soil in which our food is grown and produced. Nutrients in the soil get absorbed by the plants we eat. Yet, if the soil is lacking nutrients, which has happened in many areas due to mass agricultural practices, we also tend to lack certain nutrients.

Magnesium is also essential for adequate sleep (something many women struggle with during menopause), keeping bones strong (remember, preventing osteoporosis is key during menopause), regulating muscle and nerve function, and helping maintain balanced blood sugar levels. Some foods rich in magnesium include (chocolate lovers, rejoice!) dark chocolate, pumpkin seeds, whole grains, and beans.

IT'S NOT JUST ABOUT WHAT YOU EAT, BUT *HOW* YOU EAT

Balance is *everything*. I know this is overused but it's 110% true. We want everything in moderation to ensure we get a variety of nutrients from healthy sources. However, a good diet isn't just about *what* you eat. It's also about *how* you eat it. So, here are a few useful (and actionable) things you can keep in mind as you plan your meals and snacks.

(P.S. Planning ahead of time can make things that much easier when it comes to eating well. Consider planning your meals on your weekend and prepping as much as you can. Find a routine that works for you.).

MINDFULLY EAT & CHEW EVERY BITE FOR PAIN-FREE DIGESTION

Aim to chew each bite thoroughly. Your mouth is where digestion begins, and we want to make this process as easy as possible for our body and digestive system. Chewing every bite starts digestion, giving the stomach a bit of a break (It'll still do work but not the work it doesn't have to do) and allowing your intestines to absorb more from your food.

On top of this, don't try to distract yourself as you eat your meal or snack. Turn off the TV and put your mobile phone away. Instead, focus on the food you are eating. Taste the flavors. Enjoy your food. After all, part of the fun of eating is enjoying the flavors of the food we eat.

PAIR FOODS APPROPRIATELY FOR OPTIMAL ENERGY

Stress rises when we don't pay attention to our blood sugar levels. When we eat food, our body absorbs it, and sugar (glucose) enters the bloodstream. From there, insulin helps shuttle the sugar into the cells where it can be used for energy. The problem here is that if there isn't anything paired with the sugar or carbs you eat, then you're going to have a huge spike in your blood sugar (and energy levels) and a huge crash.

Instead of hopping on this rollercoaster ride, make sure to always eat carbs with a protein and/or fat source. This slows down the absorption of your food, giving a steady and slow supply of energy to your body as opposed to one big and quick dose. Carbs with a good fiber content, such as whole wheat options, berries, oats, and more, are also good options to slow down the digestion of your food and balance blood sugar levels.

WHAT ABOUT INTERMITTENT FASTING?

Intermittent fasting is where you eat for a set interval and fast for a set interval. There are many ways to do this, but not all apply to the menopausal woman. In fact, long fasts can wreak havoc on our hormones.

Generally, a common intermittent fasting recommendation for women during menopause is simply to fast 12-14 hours overnight. This gives your digestive system a much-needed break and won't cause adverse effects on your hormones. Studies also show improvements to weight, blood sugar, cholesterol, and blood pressure levels when intermittent fasting.

If your new to going 12-14 hours overnight without food, ease into it slowly. Simply try to space your dinner and breakfast farther apart. For instance, eat your last meal before 8 pm, then aim to have breakfast at 8 am. This gets you 12 hours of fasting!

FREQUENCY AND TIMING OF YOUR MEALS

While pairing protein, fats, and carbs together is great, you also want to space your meals appropriately throughout your day for good blood sugar regulation. When our blood sugar reduces significantly, the body actually ends up pumping out cortisol (the stress hormone) to release glucose stores in the body. This, as we explored previously, can seriously disrupt your hormones, mood, energy, symptoms, and more. In other words, we don't want the body to pump out cortisol, especially in response to low blood sugar due to not eating for hours on end. Again, planning ahead can count for a lot here when it comes to making good food choices and having healthy meals or snacks ready to eat when you need them.

PUTTING IT ALL TOGETHER...

At the end of the day, your food choices and timing of meals will all depend on your body, health, food tolerances, and lifestyle. Everyone is unique, and some may benefit from discussing their options or forming meal plans with a dietician or nutritionist. Consider figuring out your diet as a bit of an experiment. Gauge how you feel after certain foods. You may even want to keep a food journal, which involves recording how each food made you feel, until you find a good balance for you.

The general guidelines above serve as just that, guidelines. Figuring out how to make them work for you may vary when compared to others. But when you do, it's entirely worthwhile! Your diet and movement make up your foundations and offer the perfect starting point for your menopausal journey. In fact, these should come before supplements, HRT, or any of the above. Again, a combination of all of the above might work best for you. Your journey begins now.

CONCLUSION

"And for her true womanhood arrived here there is no growing old. Age refines and enriches, warms and illuminates, expands and exalts her. She is more and more Woman through it; not less and less. The noble life that has let her hither is her grand cosmetic. Her intellect, loosed from the golden bonds of corporeal Maternity, rises to the grasp of higher truths."

– Eliza W. Farnham

If you are reading this page now, you have made it to the end of the book. Did you learn something? Does this menopause "thing" now make a bit more sense now? Each of us will go through menopause in our own unique way. Your combined symptoms, whether they be physical and/or mental, will be different than what your best friend or neighbor experiences. The good news is that you have options from HRT to alternative therapies to a combination of both to exercises to food choices. The challenge and puzzle will be to figure out which of these work best for you. Hopefully after reading this book, you will have lots of information in your toolbox to make good choices and work with your healthcare providers to promote smoother sailing ahead.

The quote above is from an American novelist that lived 200 years ago. While time marches onward, the human condition remains the same while technology changes (and basically surpasses human evolution!). At the same time, Eliza's words ring so true to me. I have come out the other side of this journey and what a relief it is to no longer worry about PMS and monthly bleeding. I've experimented with HRT, alternative therapies, supplements, different exercises, and eating plans. Through trial and error, I have found what works best for my body. It was frustrating at times but worth it when I found what worked and made me feel better. We are fortunate to live in a time where we do have so many options, and this is definitely something we should emphasize and focus on.

For those in the "trenches," do not lose hope! Keep listening to your body and experimenting until you find what helps you. There is light at the end of the tunnel, no matter how long or dark your journey may seem. Getting older is a privilege that not everyone is allowed so move forward with grace, elegance, and the wisdom that you already possess.

Thank you for reading this book. If you enjoyed it, please leave a review on Amazon and spread the word.

ACKNOWLEDGEMENTS

It takes a village to write a book. It is a puzzle putting all the parts together, trying to get the ideas and topics from your head down on to paper and moulded into an informative and (hopefully) interesting book. It is especially daunting when the topic is universal and is of a scientific nature.

Thank you to Annie for your scientific knowledge. Thank you to Krista for editing this book with me. Your health expertise and wordsmithing added depth and color to my writing. Thank you to Zara for taking my ideas and making them into a beautiful book cover.

Thank you, Derek, for letting me be me and always being open to my ideas, no matter how crazy they sound.

Thank you to my mother for bringing me into this world and instilling me with a love of books and libraries.

REFERENCES

Ali, B. et al. (2015, August) Essential oils used in aromatherapy: A systemic review ScienceDirect
https://www.sciencedirect.com/science/article/pii/S2221169115001033

Baker, Fiona et al. (2019, September 1) Sleep and sleep disorders in the menopausal transition NIH: National Library of Medicine

https://www.ncbi.nlm.nih.gov/pmc/articles/PMC6092036/

Cagnacci, A and Venier, M (2019, September 18) The Controversial History of Hormone Replacement Therapy. NIH: National Library of Medicine.
https://www.ncbi.nlm.nih.gov/pmc/articles/PMC67808

Cleveland Clinic. (2021, February 18) What you should know about Chinese herbs. https://health.clevelandclinic.org/what-you-should-know-about-chinese-herbs/

Danaei, G. (2011, August 3) Bias in Observational Studies of Prevalent Users: Lessons for Comparative Effectiveness Research From a Meta-Analysis of Statins. NIH: National Library of Medicine
https://www.ncbi.nlm.nih.gov/pmc/articles/PMC3271813/

de Villiers, T.J. et al., (2016, June 20), Revised global consensus statement on menopausal hormone therapy, NIH: National Library of Medicine
https://pubmed.ncbi.nlm.nih.gov/27322027/

Fisher, P (1994, July 9) Complementary Medicine in Europe. NIH: National Library of Medicine

https://www.ncbi.nlm.nih.gov/pmc/articles/PMC2540528/pdf/bmj00448-0043.pdf

Gallagher, JC (2014) Prevention and treatment of postmenopausal osteoporosis. NIH: National Library of Medicine.

https://www.ncbi.nlm.nih.gov/pmc/articles/PMC4187361/

Geller, S. and Studee, L. (2005) Botanical and Dietary Supplements for Menopausal Symptoms: What Works, What Doesn't. NIH: National Library of Medicine.

https://www.ncbi.nlm.nih.gov/pmc/articles/PMC4187361/

Guise, Stephen (2016) Mini Habits for Weight Loss: Stop Dieting. Form New Habits. Change Your Lifestyle Without Suffering. Selective Entertainment LLC.

Gunter, J. (2021) The Menopause Manifesto: Own Your Health with Facts and Feminism. Citadel Press.

Harvard Health Publishing (2019) Menopause and Perimenopause, Take charge of the transition. Harvard Medical School. Special Health Reports.

Ho, SM. (2003, October 7) Estrogen, Progesterone and Epithelial Ovarian Cancer NIH: National Library of Medicine.

https://www.ncbi.nlm.nih.gov/pmc/articles/PMC239900/

Hongratanaworakit, T. (2006, Sept 20) Relaxing effect of ylang ylang oil on humans after transdermal absorption. NIH: National Library of Medicine. https://pubmed.ncbi.nlm.nih.gov/16807875/

Huberman, A (2021, April 12) The Science of How to Optimize Testosterone & Estrogen. Huberman Lab Podcast.

https://hubermanlab.com/the-science-of-how-to-optimize-testosterone-and-estrogen/

Jane Hailes for Women's Health (n.d) Menopause Management Options

https://www.jeanhailes.org.au/health-a-z/menopause/menopause-management

Johnson, A. (2019, March 14) Complementary and Alternative Medicine for Menopause. NIH: National Library of Medicine.

https://www.ncbi.nlm.nih.gov/pmc/articles/PMC6419242/

Jones, K. (2021, May 27) Menopause and Melatonin. The Scope. University of Utah. https://healthcare.utah.edu/the-scope/shows.php?shows=1_1jocj3fc#:~:text=It%20was%20safe%20with%20few,same%20rate%20of%20side%20effects

Kovacs, F et al. (March 1992) Experimental Study on Radioactive Pathways of Hypodermically Injected Technetium-99m Journal of Nuclear Medicine https://jnm.snmjournals.org/content/jnumed/33/3/403.full.pdf

Langer, R (2022, February 12) The women's health initiative: what can we believe? International Menopause Society podcast. https://www.youtube.com/watch?app=desktop&v=ehxlZ2Zgs7Y

Lugavere, M. (2022, October 12) The Shocking truth about menopause and how to bio hack your way through it. The Genius Life Podcast.

https://www.maxlugavere.com/podcast/256

Mayo Clinic (n.d.) Menopause: Diagnosis & Treatment. https://www.mayoclinic.org/diseases-conditions/menopause/diagnosis-treatment/drc-20353401

Medical News Today. (2022, October 26) How does menopause affect sex drive? https://www.medicalnewstoday.com/articles/320266

Merriam Webster Dictionary (n.d.). Menopause. In Merriam-Webster.com dictionary.

https://www.merriam-webster.com/dictionary/menopause

Mishra, N. (2011, Jul-Dec) Exercise beyond menopause: Dos and Don'ts.

NIH: National Library of Medicine. https://www.ncbi.nlm.nih.gov/pmc/articles/PMC3296386/

Rieck, T (2020, March 23) 10,000 steps a day: Too low? Too high? Mayo Clinic. https://www.mayoclinic.org/healthy-lifestyle/fitness/in-depth/10000-steps/art-20317391

Seol, GH (2010, July 6) Antidepressant-like effect of Salvia sclarea is explained by modulation of dopamine activities in rats. Journal of Ethnopharmacology https://www.sciencedirect.com/science/article/abs/pii/S0378874110002667

Thurlow, Cynthia (2022) Intermittent Fasting Transformation: The 45-Day Program for Women to Lose Stubborn Weight, Improve Hormonal Health, and Slow Aging. Avery.

Toffol, E. et al (2014-5) Melatonin in Perimenopausal and Postmenopausal Women. HELDA, University of Helsinki. https://helda.helsinki.fi/bitstream/handle/10138/301136/Melatonin_in_peri_and_postmenopausal_women_R1.pdf?sequence=1

Vadiveloo,M et al. (2015, March) Greater Healthful Food Variety as Measured by the US Healthy Food Diversity Index Is Associated with Lower Odds of Metabolic Syndrome and its Components in US Adults. ScienceDirect https://www.ncbi.nlm.nih.gov/pmc/articles/PMC4336534/

Vinogradova,Y. (2019, January 15) Use of hormone replacement therapy and risk of venous thromboembolism: nested case-control studies using the QResearch and CPRD databases. British Medical Journal. https://www.bmj.com/content/364/bmj.l162

Wartenberg, L. (2021) Diet and Fitness Tips for Menopause: An Essential Guide. Healthline. https://www.healthline.com/health/ten-best-menopause-activities

WebMD (n.d.) Your Guide to Menopause

http://www.webmd.com/menopause/guide/menopause-information

Wildemeersch D. (2016, August) Why perimenopausal women should consider to use a levonorgestrel intrauterine system

NIH: National Library of Medicine. https://pubmed.ncbi.nlm.nih.gov/26930021/

Zollman C. (1999, September 11) What is complementary medicine? NIH: National Library of Medicine. https://www.ncbi.nlm.nih.gov/pmc/articles/PMC1116545/

9 7 9 8 3 8 6 1 3 5 8 1 2